Biomicroscopy for Contact Lens Practice

Biomicroscopy for Contact Lens Practice: Clinical Procedures

Joe B. Goldberg, O.D., F.A.A.O.

The Professional Press, Inc.
Chicago, Illinois

All rights reserved. No part of this publication may be
reproduced or utilized in any form or by any means, electronic
or mechanical, including photocopying, recording, or any
information storage and retrieval system, without permission
in writing from the publisher, except by a reviewer who
wishes to quote brief passages in connection with a review
written for inclusion in a magazine or newspaper.

© 1970, 1984 by The Professional Press, Inc.
Second Edition 1984

ISBN 0–87873–035–4

Library of Congress Catalog Card Number
   84–62092

Published by The Professional Press, Inc.
11 E. Adams St., Suite 1209, Chicago, Illinois 60603

Printed in the U.S.A.

Dedicated to Dr. Alfred A. Rosenbloom, Jr., and the late Dr. Vincent J. Ellerbrock, without whose encouragement this book would never have been written, and to Martin Topaz, William Topaz, and Roy Stealey, whose personal interest has made it possible for this book to be published.

Table of Contents

Preface

The development of contact lenses has made it possible for vision to be corrected without conventional eyeglasses. Contact lenses are often prescribed to satisfy cosmetic needs, but they have a particular therapeutic value in the correction of such conditions as aphakia, keratoconus, keratoplasty, and low vision. Recently, they have become a sight vehicle prescribed for radial keratotomy. Their psychological importance is seen in their use as cosmetic lenses for blind or scarred eyes.

Contact lens use has increased worldwide since 1970, when the first edition of this book was published. These lenses are now accepted as primary sight vehicles by millions of people.

The concepts presented in this book are for both flexible and firm, or rigid, contact lenses. Flexible lenses are made of hydrogel or silicone elastomer materials and can be used for either daily wear or extended periods of consecutive overnight wear. Firm lenses are no longer the primary contact lens choice. However, they are prescribed for certain visual needs that cannot be satisfied with either hydrogel or silicone elastomer flexible lenses. Corneal lenses made of gas-permeable materials are gradually replacing those made of polymethylmethacrylate (PMMA).

Chapter 1 describes the role of biomicroscopy in contact lens practice. It shows the historical development of the biomicroscope and explains how the principles of biomicroscopy are applied to contact lens fitting. Chapter 2 discusses the basic design of the biomicroscope, the phenomenon of reflection as it affects the cornea, and the techniques of biomicroscope examination and photography. Chapter 3 reviews corneal anatomy and physiology, emphasizing the importance of corneal transparency. Chapter 4 presents the practical applications of biomicroscopy. Chapter 5 is a conspectus on fitting hydrogel contact lenses. It describes how biomicroscopy is used to fit these lenses for daily and extended wear. Chapters 6 and 7 deal with firm corneal lenses, including the use of biomicroscopy in determining lens modifications. Chapter 8 concludes the book with a description of silicone elastomer contact lenses and of the use of biomicroscopes in fitting them.

In the early years of contact lens development, one could easily describe contact lens fitting with the maxim *caveat emptor*. Today, we can proudly exclaim *"tempora mutantur"* (times are changed). No longer is it necessary to seek contact lens fitting instruction only from private sources or to rely exclusively on manufacturers' fitting manuals. The growth and maturity of contact lens practice is reflected in the academic and clinical programs at all optometry schools, in ophthalmological residencies, in continuing education courses sponsored by optometric and medical groups, and in the various contact lens textbooks now available.

Successful contact lens fitting is directly related to the practitioner's skill and knowledge of biomicroscopy as a clinical technique. In preparing this text, I have attempted to distill the knowledge and experience gathered in more than 30 years of service to contact lens patients. It is my hope that the information presented here will help both students and contact lens practitioners in their use of biomicroscopy to fit contact lenses.

Acknowledgments

Often, writing a book requires the coordinated skills and knowledge of several people; one person alone may travel a path of exasperation and confusion, wading through what seems an endless amount of material. Although the author assumes the responsibility for the actual writing, others have read, criticized, and made suggestions about the book.

I want to thank Dr. Roger Cummings for updating the information in Chapter 2 on biomicroscope instruments and photography.

I would also like to thank Dr. Joseph T. Barr, Dr. Edward S. Bennett, Dr. Neil Hodur, and Dr. Alfred A. Rosenbloom, Jr., for their evaluations and suggestions.

I want to express my appreciation to Laura Alman, my editorial consultant, and to Dr. Leonard Werner, the publisher's liaison.

I am also indebted to thousands of contact lens patients for their unquestioning allegiance during my formative and recent years in contact lens practice, and I thank them for agreeing to sit patiently while I took an unlimited number of biomicroscope photographs.

Joe B. Goldberg, O.D., F.A.A.O.

Chapter 1

Biomicroscopy and Contact Lens Practice

Contact lens fitting has made many practitioners aware of biomicroscopy and has emphasized the need for its use. Biomicroscopy is the examination of the living eye by means of an instrument that consists of both a controlled illumination source, often called a slit lamp, and a corneal microscope. Biomicroscopy can be considered an intravital, histologic method for studying the ocular tissues.[1]

Prior to the acceptance of contact lens fitting, the biomicroscope was used only in medical diagnosis. Now, however, it is considered a necessary piece of objective instrumentation that is vital to the effectiveness of contact lens practice procedures.

Using biomicroscopy for contact lens fitting, one can observe conditions of poor lacrimal interchange, constant bearing areas, epithelial disturbances, and areas of incipient vascularization that may not be detectable with lesser degrees of illumination and magnification. No system in use today can equal the effectiveness of the magnification and illumination provided by the biomicroscope.

The contact lens practitioner using the biomicroscope will receive guidance concerning the effectiveness of the lens design for the patient and will be stimulated to achieve greater accuracy in creating all contact lens design components. With biomicroscopy, the contact lens practitioner will be secure in the knowledge that the design will not interfere with the prerequisites for maintaining corneal transparency. The biomicroscope will help the practitioner decide whether to change or retain any or all of the contact lens design components and will facilitate the prescribing of specialized contact lens designs and materials (for example, small, thin, steep, gas-permeable corneal contact lenses; noncircular designs; hydrogel, silicone, and silicone organic copolymer firm contact lens materials).

Gross, naked-eye surveys of the contact lens fit are not to be eliminated; nor is it suggested that the established black-light and fluorescein technique be discarded. Instead, it is suggested that these techniques be classified as additional procedures to be used prior to biomicroscopy.

The biomicroscope is an invaluable ally for pre–contact lens

1

fitting information. It furnishes information related to corneal structure (corneal dystrophy, superficial placement of corneal nerves, and quality of conjunctival tissue formations, vessels adjacent to the cornea, and their extension on it, for example) that could influence any decision for prescribing contact lenses. In fact, Doggart[2] has stated that only the biomicroscope can detect Fuchs's dystrophy, since this condition involves the disintegration of the endothelial mosaic.

The biomicroscope serves as an excellent guide in all phases of contact lens service—from the period of patient selection through the fitting period, culminating in the individual post-care program. The ability to vary the intensity of illumination and the direction of the beam of light makes this a significant instrument for evaluating the cornea during contact lens wear.

When one uses an applanation tonometer in conjunction with the biomicroscope, the latter's value is enhanced. Also, one may employ the biomicroscope as a binocular ophthalmoscope for indirect ophthalmoscopy by using (1) a contact lens having a flat anterior surface so that the corneal refraction is eliminated and a virtual image of the fundus is produced in the anterior segment of the eye, (2) a strong concave lens (Hruby lens) attached to the instrument and placed in position directly in front of and a short distance from the cornea so that a focus can be obtained on the fundus, and (3) a strong convex lens placed in front of the cornea to form a real inverted image of the fundus between it and the miscroscope.[3]

HISTORICAL DEVELOPMENT OF BIOMICROSCOPY

In 1891 Aubert presented a binocular corneal microscope at the Ophthamological Congress in Heidelberg.[4] Czapski[5] modified the Aubert corneal microscope, and Zeiss added refinements that made the Czapski-Zeiss corneal microscope better: An erect image with a full stereoscopic effect was obtained by a system of Porro prisms with four reflections, and the eyepieces could be adjusted to suit the interpupillary distance of the examiner. However, the value of this microscope was not fully established until Alvar Gullstrand[6] solved the problem of illumination. The design of all subsequent corneal microscopes has been based on these principles.

Prior to Gullstrand's invention, a system of lens and loupe was used; in it, a biconvex lens formed an oblique beam on the eye from a nearby lamp. Wolff first used a carbon filament bulb ophthalmoscope, with light passing through a condensing lens, being reflected into the eye by means of an oblique mirror, and casting an image of the filament on the retina.[7] This was the first truly focused beam for the examination of oscular tissue.

In 1911 Gullstrand presented the first rudimentary model of the slit lamp to the German ophthalmologists in Heidelberg. It was the first time a satisfactory method of examining the anterior parts of the living eye was made available. The Nernst lamp served as the basis for illumination. Its filament was composed of a tightly coiled tungsten spiral, coated with a compound of metallic oxides that became incandescent when electrified. The lamp was rod shaped and therefore suitable for use with a slit diaphragm. Gullstrand developed a method for projecting the image of the Nernst rod in a slit opening to produce a rectangular focal beam. The model of the Nernst slit lamp illuminating unit constructed in 1908 was used originally to measure the posterior corneal surface. In 1909 it was used at the Uppsala Clinic (Stockholm) as a source of focal illumination for examining the transparent ocular media.

Gullstrand projected the rays of light emanating from an image of the light source rather than those emitted by the luminous body itself, thus making it possible to obtain a controllable beam of strongly focused light without the disadvantage of ordinary oblique illumination.

In 1916 Henker mounted Gullstrand's illuminating system on a horizontal rigid swinging arm in conjunction with the Czapski corneal microscope. This modification permitted relative steadiness as well as mobility so that a more detailed examination of the eye could be made. The light that fell on the part of the eye to be examined was an image of an image. The Nernst filament's image was focused on the slit, and an image from this slit enclosed image was in turn directed on the eye. Both images were of uniform light because the filament was homogeneous.

When the Nernst lamp became unavailable after World War I, Gullstrand used the Nitra bulb, which was constructed by winding tungsten in a container filled with nitrogen. Because the Nitra bulb did not furnish uniform light, Gullstrand made several clinical adjustments in his technique. Vogt made the next major change in the lamp's design by moving the lamp forward so that homogeneous light filled the slit and the illumination was increased. This modification led to the development of the narrow beam of direct illumination (optical section). Later refinements were made by Koeppe, Koby, Lopez-Lacarrere, Comberg, Arruga, Poser, and others.

THE PRINCIPLES OF BIOMICROSCOPY APPLIED TO CONTACT LENS PRACTICE

Biomicroscopy depends on the full use of the focal illumination (light projected by a condensing lens or a series of lenses). At the focal point of such a system the light becomes intensely concentrated. Gullstrand's system, as modified by Vogt, makes it possible to examine the successive layers of the transparent ocular media illuminated by light in exact focus.

The small section of tissues illuminated by the focused light as it passes through the transparent media of the eye corresponds to the size and shape of the beam. There is a marked contrast between the illuminated area and the surrounding area in shadow. This effect, comparable to that of a searchlight beam passing through the sky, is called the *Tyndall phenomenon*. In 1868 Tyndall used floating dust to reveal the paths of luminous beams through the air. Suspended particles are made visible when one directs an intense beam of light across the field of the objective at angles to the axis of the microscope. Each particle scatters some of this light; the scattered light, which enters the objective from any one particle, is focused as a diffraction disc in the image plane of the microscope ocular, becoming visible to the eye by means of increased intensities of light and the apparent increase in size obtained by the formation of diffraction discs.

The cornea, lens, and vitreous exhibit the Tyndall phenomenon in varying degrees. The phenomenon becomes more apparent in pathological conditions.

The normal cornea is avascular, laminated, and transparent. The biophysical and biochemical properties of the cornea and the type of insult determine the nature of corneal reaction. Staining of the precorneal film line with fluorescein assists in the exact localization of insult. It also reveals any break that may have occurred on the corneal epithelium. Corneal lesions may or may not be accompanied by vascular invasion. In contact lens practice we are primarily and immediately concerned with epithelial staining. Normally, the epithelial surface is protected by the fluid of the precorneal film line. Any condition that prevents normal physiologic passage of fluids or gases through the epithelium causes stasis and resultant epithelial edema.

When the epithelium is abraded, it is loosened. The insult may be superficial or may become subepithelial. Fluorescein staining may create the impression that the stainable section is larger than it actually is. Attention should therefore be given to the anterior surface of the stained precorneal film line, since danger may arise from possible infection through the exposed corneal section. An epithelial structural alteration indicates that the controls for the water balance of the cornea and its gaseous exchange are in need of repair.

The biomicroscope becomes a valuable asset in contact lens practice because with it one can objectively observe areas of poor contact lens design and their immediate effect on the cornea's prerequisites for maintaining transparency and can make contact lens design modification before corneal insult develops to any degree. Thus, one may consider biomicroscopy as an objective control method for observing and accumulating data related to the effectiveness of a contact lens design.

NOTES

1. M. L. Berliner, *Biomicroscopy of the Eye* (London: Hamish Hamilton Medical Books, 1949).

2. J. H. Doggart, *Ocular Signs in Slit-Lamp Microscopy* (St. Louis: C. V. Mosby, 1949).

3. S. Duke-Elder, ed., *System of Ophthalmology,* vol. 7 (St. Louis: C. V. Mosby, 1962).

4. Berliner, *Biomicroscopy of the Eye.*

5. S. Czapski, "Binocular Corneal Mikroskop," *Archives of Ophthalmology* 48 (1899); 229–235.

6. A. Gullstrand, "Demonstration der Nernstspatlampe," *Berichte über die Versammlungen der deutschen ophthalmologischen Gesellschaft* 37 (1911): 374.

7. Berliner, *Biomicroscopy of the Eye.*

Chapter 2

Basic Design of the Modern Biomicroscope and Biomicroscope Photography

Roger Cummings
Contributing Author

The evolution of the biomicroscope has progressed since the slit lamp of Gullstrand[1] was combined with the microscope invented by Czapski.[2] Subsequent improvements have allowed the microscope and slit lamp to be mounted so that they are cofocal. All modern biomicroscopes allow full movement of either the illumination source or the observation system; neither interferes with the other. Modern biomicroscopes also incorporate a joy stick mechanism that allows rapid and accurate positioning of the instrument.

All modern slit lamp biomicroscopes are composed of four important components: (1) a horizontally mounted binocular microscope, (2) an incandescent light source with filters and mirrors to control illumination, (3) an instrument positioning mechanism to control movement of the instrument, and (4) a patient positioning system incorporating a headrest and fixation target. Most modern biomicroscopes also have certain accessories that are invaluable for complete examination of the eye. Among them are applanation tonometers to determine intraocular pressure and Hruby lenses to observe the fundus and posterior vitreous. In addition, some biomicroscopes allow teaching tubes, pachometers, and photographic accessories to be added onto the basic instrument. It is important to evaluate these accessories with regard to the needs of contact lens practice, since accessories that interfere with the observation and manipulation of a contact lens will make the examination more difficult than it should be.

Certain important features of each of these components will be examined here. There are two basic microscope systems, each

Roger Cummings, O.D., F.A.A.O., is an associate professor at the Pennsylvania College of Optometry and a staff optometrist at its Eye Institute.

Figure 2-1. American Optical Campbell biomicroscope. Courtesy of American Optical Corporation.

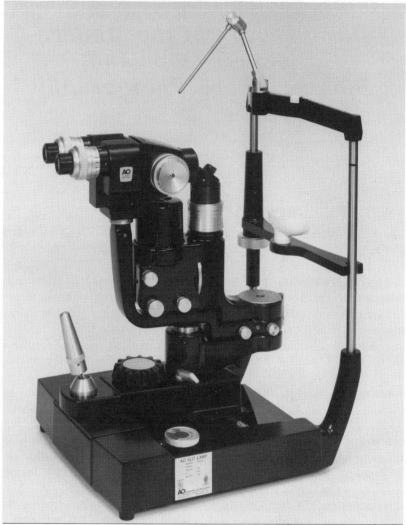

having certain advantages and disadvantages. The one developed by Haag-Streit for its Universal 900 consists of an optical system with converging axes. Magnification is controlled by a lever operated turret system that aligns different objectives in the optical path. It can be changed by replacing the oculars. Topcon, Marco, and Mentor produce similar microscopes. The advantages of this system are compactness, low light loss through the optical system, and ease in attaining stereopsis. The disadvantages are a limited range

Figure 2–2. Bausch & Lomb biomicroscope. Courtesy of Bausch & Lomb Corporation.

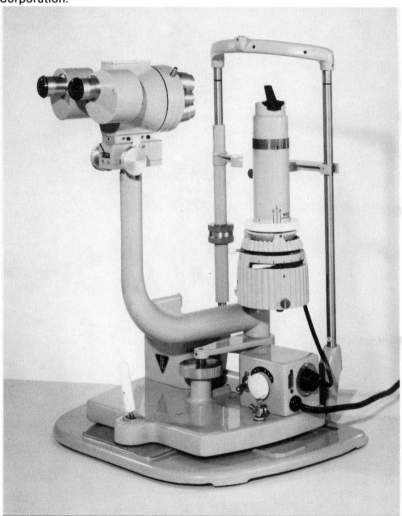

of magnification before the need to change the oculars and the difficulty of adding accessories. The second major type of microscope system involves a Galilean telescope placed between the primary and secondary objectives. This type of system, developed by Zeiss, is also used in the American Optical Campbell and Topcon SL–5D. Its advantages are a wide range of magnifications without changing oculars and extreme flexibility in adding observation tubes and photographic accessories. This system will produce a slight loss in

Figure 2–3. Haag-Streit Universal Model 900 biomicroscope. Courtesy of Haag-Streit AG.

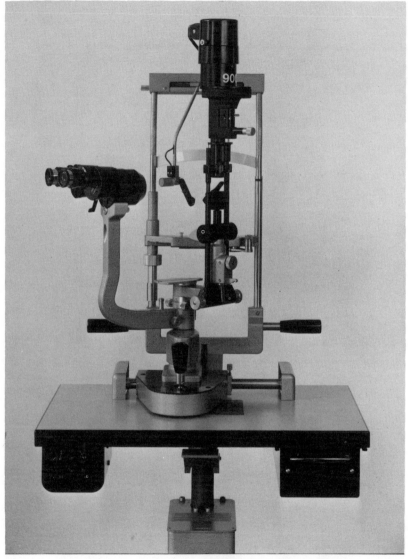

light transmission at higher magnifications and when beam splitters are interposed to allow the use of the observation tubes or to photograph some ocular structure.

The illumination system of the biomicroscope, developed from Gullstrand's original slit lamp, allows a sharply focused beam to be coincident with the focus of the microscope. Of particular impor-

Figure 2–4. Haag-Streit Standard Model 900 biomicroscope, a simplified version of the Universal Model 900. This model does not have the turret that allows a magnification change of the objectives. In addition, the illumination system does not adjust to change the inclination of the beam. Courtesy of Haag-Streit AG.

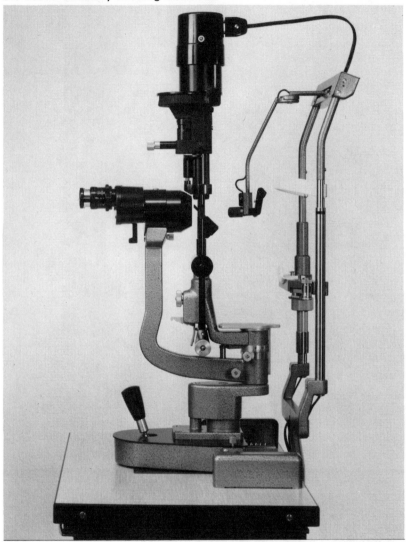

tance to contact lens examinations is the use of a blue filter to heighten the visibility of fluorescein after it has been instilled in the tear film. This filter can be quickly interposed in all biomicroscopes described in this chapter.

There are two major variations on the illumination systems

Figure 2–5. Photographic attachment for Haag-Streit biomicroscope. Courtesy of Haag-Streit AG.

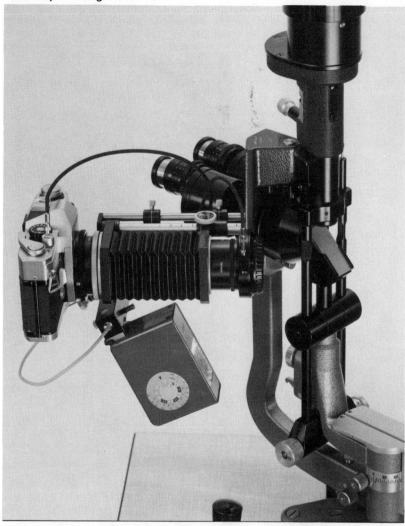

in modern biomicroscopes. The vertically oriented illumination system, developed by Haag-Streit, features an incandescent bulb mounted at the top of the illumination system; a variety of filters are interposed before the mirror, which reflects the light beam toward the patient. Another valuable feature is the micrometer control of slit height, which allows a direct reading of the size of an object. Similar illumination systems are found in Topcon, Marco, and Mentor biomicroscopes. The other major illumination system, developed by Zeiss, uses several prisms to divert the light from

Figure 2–6. Marco IIb biomicroscope. Courtesy of Marco Ophthalmic Instuments.

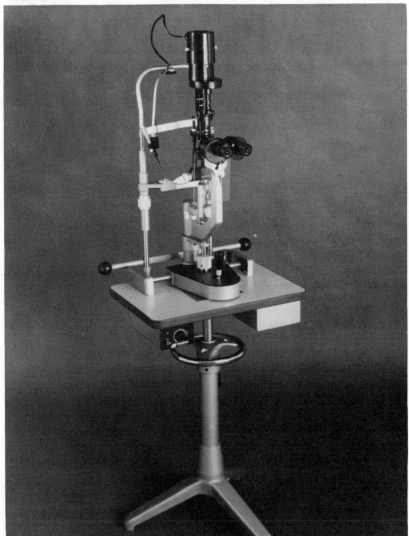

the incandescent source toward the patient. American Optical, Bausch & Lomb, and Nikon use similar systems for their slit lamp sources.

The design of the illumination system should allow for easy manipulation of the various controls and should prevent dust from collecting on the surfaces of the optical elements. In addition, stray light should not fall on the patient's eye, since this can obscure such corneal conditions as corneal edema. Finally, adjustments to control the inclination of the slit beam, such as the tilting mechanism in the Haag-Streit Universal 900 and the prism control in the Zeiss Model 30, have little purpose in contact lens practice. Their use in gonioscopy and fundus and vitreous examination is fully described by Tolentino, Schepens, and Freeman.[3]

MODERN BIOMICROSCOPE PHOTOGRAPHY

Most major biomicroscope manufacturers offer some photographic attachments for their instruments. For contact lens practice the basic biomicroscope design must not be compromised, since the instrument will be used primarily for examinations, not photography. The photographic accessories should be fully integrated into the instrument design and should allow immediate use of the camera. The biomicroscope and accessories should be compact enough to allow for routine manipulation of the patient's eyes and contact lenses.

True slit lamp photography requires extremely bright light from the slit beam to provide adequate film exposure, especially for photographs requiring a fine slit. With present film sensitivity, this light can be provided only by an electronic flash tube mounted in the slit beam optical section, usually between the incandescent light source and the slit beam controls. In this way, the slit characteristics will be duplicated in the photograph. Provision is usually made for a second accessory flash for fill-in illumination. This flash provides illumination of the surrounding ocular structures, which aids in orienting the final photograph. Successful slit lamp photographs require the balancing of these two flash sources. Since photographic film is far less tolerant than the human eye of differences in illumination level, the balance of light sources is more critical than in routine biomicroscopy. In addition, since still photography records one point in time, the viewer of the photograph does not have the benefit of integrating different views over the course of the biomicroscopic examination. For these reasons, slit lamp photography remains very much an art. Some of the difficulties in exposure may be reduced in the future if electronic metering systems capable of controlling electronic flash duration are incorporated into photo slit lamps. This feature, which could be most effective at the film plane, already exists in one 35 mm camera for general photography.

Certain photographic guidelines can be followed to help the practitioner take acceptable photographs through the biomicroscope. Magnification should be set higher than that normally used for examination procedures, because the camera body is positioned between the objective and the ocular lens of the biomicroscope and therefore does not benefit from the final magnification from the

Figure 2–7. Marco III biomicroscope. This model features an inclination control for the illumination system. Courtesy of Marco Ophthalmic Instruments.

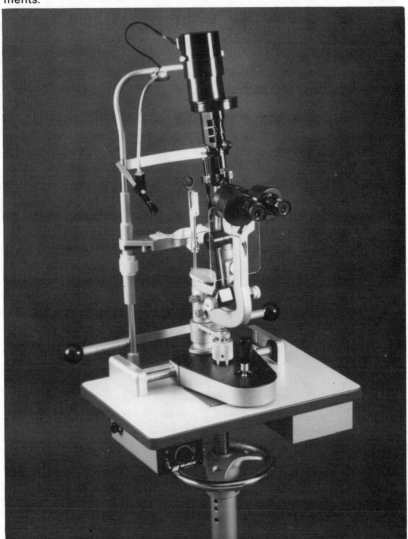

ocular lens. Slit lamp photographs are most valuable at magnifications of 1.6x to 2.5x. This magnification corresponds to settings of 16x or 25x with 10x oculars. In general, as magnification is increased, the output of the electronic flash unit must be increased. This is especially true for optical systems with Galilean telescopes interposed between the objectives. Ocular tissues have very different reflective characteristics. White scleral tissue reflects a great deal

Figure 2–8. Marco V–P Photo slit lamp biomicroscope. This model features an elevation control concentric to the joy stick. Courtesy of Marco Ophthalmic Instruments.

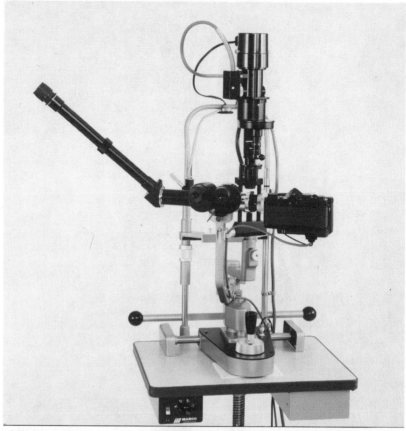

of light; optical sections of transparent media reflect little light.

The Zeiss photo slit lamp, introduced in 1965, was a major advancement in biomicroscope photography. It was the first instrument to contain an electronic flash in the optical path of the illumination system. This advancement allowed true slit beam photographs to be taken. In addition, a fill-in flash illuminated surrounding ocular tissue so that proper orientation of the structure could be appreciated. The Zeiss photo slit lamp allowed the mounting of one or two camera bodies on the microscope, which meant that true slit lamp stereo photographs could be taken simultaneously. A more recent innovation is the Urban stereo adaptor, which allows simultaneous stereo photographs to be produced on one 35 mm film frame. Unfortunately, the Zeiss photo slit lamp is bulky, and the distance from the oculars to the patient is sufficiently long to make manipulation of the lids or lenses difficult.

Figure 2-9. Nikon photo slit lamp biomicroscope. Courtesy of Nikon Ophthalmic Instruments.

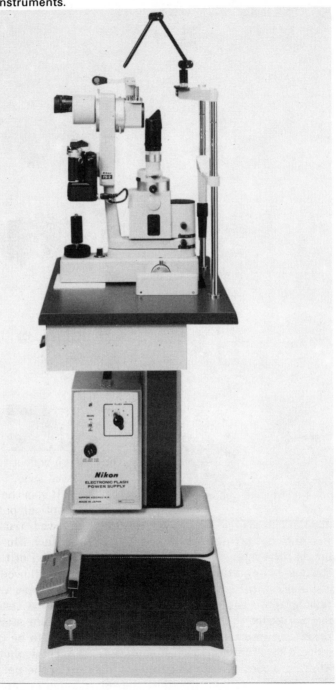

Figure 2–10. Topcon SL–2D biomicroscope. Courtesy of Topcon Instrument Corporation.

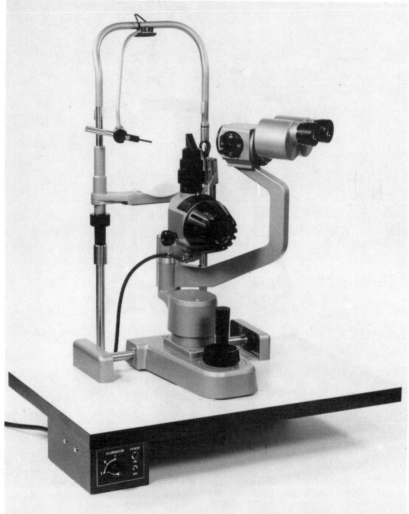

In addition, the instrument is heavy and must therefore be mounted on its own table. These characteristics detract from it utility in routine examinations.

A significant step toward providing practitioners with slit lamp photographic equipment is the Nikon photo slip lamp—the first biomicroscope to allow true slit lamp photography at a reasonable price. The optical system of the instrument consists of a zoom microscope whose magnification is continuously variable from 7x to 35x. There are convenient click stops at 10x, 16x, and 25x. The camera

Figure 2–11. Topcon SL–3D biomicroscope. Courtesy of Topcon Instrument Corporation.

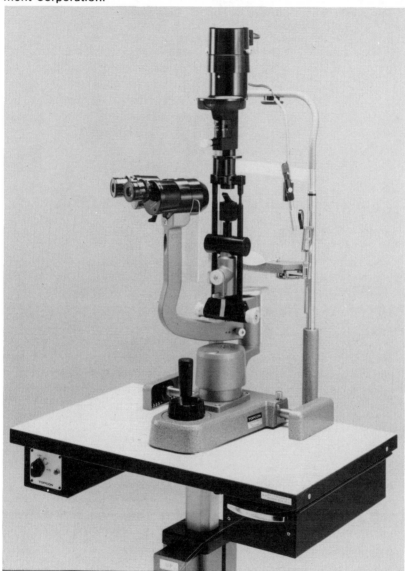

body is well integrated into the microscope optics. A tube extends from the upper side of the microscope, and the Nikon or Nikkormat camera body fits onto the top of the tube. When a picture is taken, the operator lowers a flange on this tube, which allows a mirror to direct the image away from the ocular to the camera body. Thus, the view through the ocular is blocked during the time the picture

Figure 2–12. Topcon SL–5D photo slit lamp biomicroscope. This model has a Galilean telescope and beam splitter incorporated into the design of the microscope. Courtesy of Topcon Instrument Corporation.

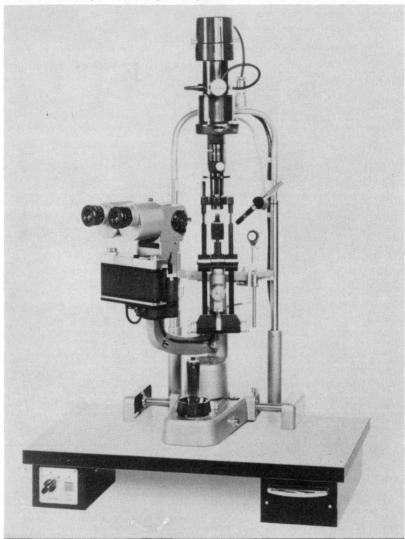

is taken. The advantage of this mirror system is that it allows full illumination to the ocular until the picture is taken and full illumination to the camera body when the picture is taken.

The illumination system of the Nikon biomicroscope is positioned under the line of sight of the microscope; it is controlled by a variety of prisms, lenses, and filters. Just as in the Zeiss photo slit lamp, the gas discharge tube is placed in the focused beam of

Figure 2–13. Zeiss 30SL biomicroscope. All Zeiss biomicroscopes allow the addition of a beam splitter and photographic tube for external ocular photography. Courtesy of Carl Zeiss, Incorporated.

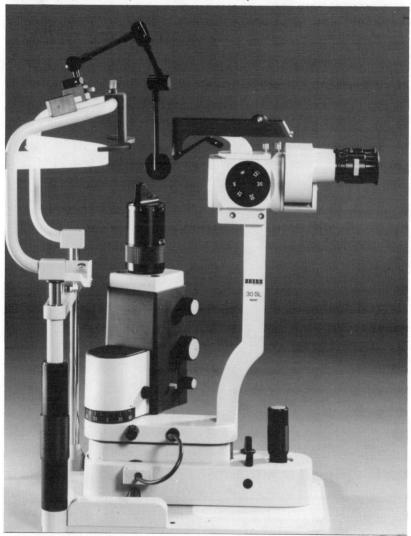

the incandescent light source, thus providing true slit lamp photographs. In addition to the usual slit lamp controls, the Nikon photo slit lamp has an iris diaphragm to diminish the intensity of the light and a unique continuous control of slit height and width that allows for quick adjustment of the illuminating beam. The Nikon does not come equipped with a fill-in flash like that of the Zeiss unit. Instead, Nikon uses a diffusing filter, placed in the filter holder

Figure 2–14. Zeiss 30SL biomicroscope with photographic attachment. Courtesy of Carl Zeiss, Incorporated.

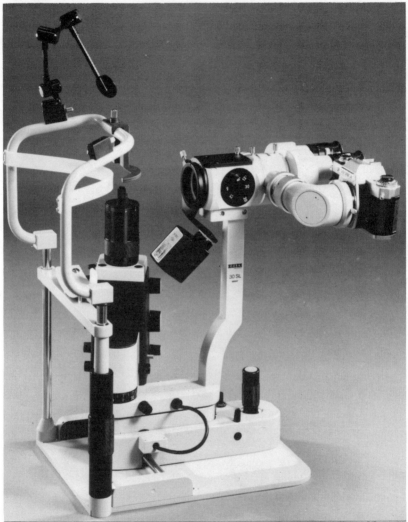

of the illuminating system, to achieve fill-in illumination. This system produces satisfactory photographs at higher magnifications if a medium to wide beam is used to illuminate the subject.

If a fine beam is used, the filter provides little fill-in illumination. To overcome this problem, an inexpensive external strobe light can be used to control the fill-in illumination.[4] In this case, a Vivitar flash unit is attached with a straight and swivel bracket to the tripod socket of the camera body.

Figure 2–15. Nikon photo slit lamp with strobe light attachment to control fill-in illumination. Courtesy of Nikon Ophthalmic Instruments.

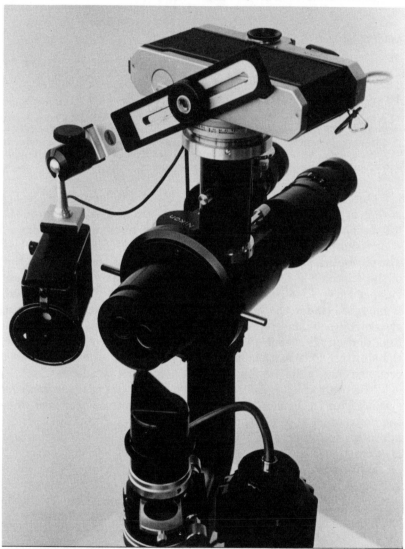

For photography, the intensity of the slit lamp beam is controlled by a five-step capacitor. Kaps,[5] Rengstorff and Krause,[6] and Spivak[7] offer suggestions for using this control to obtain the proper exposure for slit lamp photographs. Spivak's suggestions are reproduced in Table 2–1. They are only guidelines, however; excellent photographs are produced by proper adjustments or by bracketing the suggested exposures.

Table 2-1 Suggested Aperture Size for Proper Exposure at Various Magnifications with Two Commonly Available Film Speeds[a]

	Aperture Size	
Magnification	ASA 200 film	ASA 400 film
35×	5.5, 7.0, 8.0, 9.5	5.0, 5.5, 7.0, 8.0
25×	5.5, 7.0	5.0, 5.5
16×	5.0, 5.5	4.0, 5.0
10×	4.0, 5.0	4.0

[a] Recommended film for color transparencies is Kodak High-Speed Ektrachrome (ASA 200), and for black and white photographs is Kodak Tri-X (ASA 400). A smaller aperture size will allow underexposure of fill-in flash. Selective underexposure is desirable at high magnification (35×) because of flare produced by the microscope optics.

One of the most advanced designs in slit lamp photography is that of the Topcon Instrument Corporation. The Topcon SL–5D microscope system incorporates a Galilean telescope that allows a wide magnification range without the need to change the oculars. The slit optics are arranged vertically, in a manner similar to that of the Topcon SL–3 and the Haag-Streit. The photographic accessories are exceptionally well designed and compact. The camera body is mounted under the microscope and is connected to the viewing system by a beam splitter. A compact autowinder advances the film, and an electronic switch on the top of the joy stick activates the shutter. This feature is especially valuable when one hand is occupied manipulating the patient's lids or contact lenses.

The beam splitter can be switched into or out of the microscope system. This feature enables a brighter image to be projected when the instrument is used for routine biomicroscopic examination and allows an uninterrupted view of the patient when the photograph is taken.

A five-position capacitor controls the flash discharge tube, which is imaged in the slit beam optical path. A fiber optic bundle diverts some of the flash to serve as diffuse fill-in illumination. Two apertures control this illumination. In certain situations, additional fill-in illumination may produce a better photograph. This illumination can be provided by an accessory flash similar to that for the Nikon photo slit lamp.[8]

The Marco photo slit lamps (Models IIB–P and V–P) offer some important features for slit lamp photography. The microscope system has converging optics, which allows easier fusion of the two images. Magnification changes of 1x or 1.6x are provided by a rapid internal change of the objectives. Magnifications of 2x and 3.2x are available with an optional teleplus lens. The beam splitter is positioned between the objectives and the oculars of the instrument, which allows a continuous view of the eye even while the photograph is being taken.

The camera body can be mounted on the left or right side of the instrument to correspond with the view from either eye. The mounting arm of the camera body has an adjustable aperture diaphragm corresponding to f-stops of 1.0, 1.4, 2.0, 2.8, 4.0, and 5.6. This control allows for adjustment of the light level and depth of focus in the photograph. The suggested camera body is Olympus OM–1 with motor drive. The shutter release for the camera is connected to the joy stick of the instrument. This feature allows the practitioner to use one hand to adjust the position of the patient's lids or contact lenses while the other hand controls the focusing and shutter release.

The illumination system is vertically arranged and allows a wide variation of filters and other controls on the slit beam. The flash discharge tube is positioned between the incandescent bulb and the remainder of the illuminating system. It is controlled by a five-step capacitor. In addition, a 5 mm fiber optic illuminator provides fill-in illumination for photography.

Both the Marco and Topcon SL–5D photo slit lamps provide significant advantages for practitioners doing slit lamp photography. They offer a convenient working distance, their photographic accessories have been well integrated into the overall design of the biomicroscope, and their fiber optic illuminators provide some additional exposure of the surrounding ocular structures without the complexity of a separate fill-in flash. Finally, the joy stick mounted shutter control is an important advance for convenience in obtaining slit lamp photographs.

The photographic attachment for the Haag-Streit slit lamp consists of a 35 mm camera body, bellows unit, macro lens, and external flash. A bracket connects the camera body to a mounting rod over the microscope objectives. This is the same mounting rod on which the tonometer may be positioned; therefore, these two accessories cannot be used at the same time. The system is essentially the same as the ones described for external ocular photography,[9] but it allows the use of the joy stick focusing and the headrest of the Haag-Streit biomicroscope.

NOTES

1.   A. Gullstrand, "Demonstration der Nernstspatlampe," *Berichte über die Versammlungen der deutschen ophthalmologischen Gesselschaft* 37 (1911): 374.

2.   S. Czapski, "Binoculares Corneal Mikroskop," *Archives of Ophthalmology* 48 (1899): 229–235.

3.   F. Tolentino, C. Schepens, and H. Freeman, *Vitreoretinal Disorders: Diagnosis and Management* (Philadelphia: W. B. Saunders, 1976): pp. 71–108.

4.   R. Cummings, R. Clompus, and R. Ellis, "An Accessory Flash for the Nikon Photo Slit Lamp," *American Journal of Optometry and Physiological Optics* 56 (1979): 128–132.

5.   S. Kaps. "Slit-Lamp Photography," *Optical Journal and Review of Optometry* 107 (1970): 41–54.

6.   R. Rengstorff and C. Krause, "Guide for Slit Lamp Photography of the Cornea," *American Optometric Association Journal* 42 (1971): 1250–1255.

7.   T. Spivak, "Photography through the Nikon Slit Lamp Biomicroscope," *Review of Optometry* 114 (1977): 56–60.

8.   Cummings, Clompus, and Ellis, *Accessory Flash.*

9.   K. Cuiffreda, "Understanding Fluorescein Contact Lens Photography," *American Optometric Association Journal* 46 (1975): 706–713; R. Guther, "Anterior Segment Photography," *American Optometric Association Journal* 48 (1977): 41–45.

Chapter 3

Corneal Transparency and Contact Lenses

Besides the obvious necessity for corneal transparency to support the human optical system, the fact that the cornea is transparent affords us the unique opportunity to observe, with the aid of a biomicroscope, the condition of all the layers of corneal tissue in vivo. Since pathological changes in the various corneal layers (either before contact lens wear or induced by contact lenses) can affect corneal transparency, it is important that we understand the properties that make the cornea unique.

François and Rabaey[1] emphasized that corneal transparency is dependent on the microscopic corneal framework and the concentration of histochemical and ultramicroscope structure. Phase contrast microscopy, historadiography, and electron microscopy provide an understanding of the interrelationship of the factors responsible for the maintenance of corneal transparency. Interestingly, a very cloudy cornea sometimes shows only slight histological changes.

The lattice theory of corneal transparency proposed by Maurice[2] is based on the regular arrangement of the corneal fibrillae. The fibrillae are uniform, equal in diameter, and arranged in a regular two-dimensional lattice formation.[3] Maurice compared the fibrillae to a diffraction grating where scratches are very close to each other, the spacing less than the wavelength of light. Under this condition, there is very little scattering of light, except in the direction of the incident beam, and the cornea appears to be transparent. Corneal swelling causes the rows of fibrillae to separate from each other, which results in a disorderly arrangement and loss of corneal transparency. A swelling of the mucoid in which the fibrillae are embedded can cause cloudiness by light scatter.

In discussing corneal transparency, Davson[4] referred to the manner in which light is transmitted by a material rather than the ability of a material to transmit light. Describing the perfect optical image created by dark glasses, which may reduce the transmission to 10 percent of the incident intensity, he compared the glasses with an opal screen, which may reduce the intensity less than glasses do but which precludes the formation of an image because of the scattering of the light. Davson concluded that the cornea is transparent because less than 1 percent of the light is scattered.

Since corneal swelling is associated with a loss of corneal transparency, the design dimensions of the contact lens must not cause it to impinge on an area associated with the oxygen supply requirements for the eye. Metabolic energy is necessary for maintaining corneal thickness, and any absence or reduction in the amount of oxygen necessary for supplying this energy will create an increase in corneal thickness and result in the fogging of vision.[5]

Cogan and Kinsey[6] suggested that the cornea remains transparent because the limiting layers of the cornea act as semipermeable membranes and an osmotic difference across them counters the swelling pressure of the stroma. The osmotic difference results from the secretion of an aqueous humor hypertonic blood and therefore hypertonic to the stroma, which is in equilibrium with the blood.

Disagreeing with this hypothesis, Maurice[7] commented that the proposed mechanism does not appear to be feasible. He stated that the endothelium is permeable to the important solute of the aqueous humor and that the cornea apparently is able to maintain the difference in osmotic pressure by the action of its own metabolism. According to Maurice, the epithelium and endothelium are themselves barriers to water transfer. Maurice considered this point significant. He stated that the resistance exists only in the epithelium, not in Bowman's layer, and that it is probably in the epithelial surface layer since this layer is very sensitive to the touch. The resistance present in the endothelium does not occur in Descemet's membrane either.

Adler[8] described the metabolic activity of the cornea as involving respiration and glycolysis. Respiration, which takes place mainly in the epithelium, requires the presence of oxygen and results in the production of carbon dioxide and water and the liberation of energy. The liberated energy is available for cellular activity and for maintenance of tissue temperature. Glycolysis may take place in either the presence or absence of oxygen and in either the epithelium or the stroma.

The sources of an adequate oxygen supply to the cornea are the precorneal fluid, the limbal capillaries, the aqueous humor, and oxygen from the atmosphere. The precorneal fluid furnishes oxygen to the cornea and helps carry away metabolic waste materials. A contact lens may reduce or obstruct the lacrimal flow in areas of corneal bearing and may create a decrease in the oxygen supply furnished by both the precorneal fluid and the limbal capillaries. As a result, there is (1) an increase in lactic acid, (2) interference with corneal gaseous exchange requirements, and (3) formation underneath the contact lens of carbon dioxide bubbles that create pressure against the corneal epithelial surface and cause corneal epithelial edema in restricted local areas.

When the epithelial surface is no longer a barrier to the invasion of water into the cornea and the contact lens design is not modified in situ, the condition worsens. The edema induced in the epithelium may spread to the deeper corneal layers and cause severe corneal damage.

The epithelium is important for carbohydrate metabolism of the cornea. In the epithelium, glucose is broken down into lactic acid; and although lactic acid cannot be oxidized further by the stroma, further oxidation can take place in the epithelium, where a complete system exists for the oxidation of glucose into carbon dioxide and water.

Ashton[9] described the cornea as being avascular and as having sluggish circulation and minimal oxygen supply. He reported that lactic acid concentration in the cornea decreases when the oxygen tension in the tear fluid increases. The cornea produces lactic acid at a high rate whenever the oxygen supply to the cornea is insufficient to maintain maximal respiration.

Smelser and Chen[10] reported that the concentration of lactic acid increases as a function of the time during which an improperly fitted contact lens is worn. They found a decrease in corneal transparency coincident with the rise in lactic acid concentration.

Hirano[11] observed a widening of the intercellular spaces, disarrangement of corneal epithelial cells, thickening of the stroma, dilatation of iris vessels, and changes in glycogen when an improperly fitted contact lens was worn. These findings show that a proper glycogen reserve must be maintained by adequate precorneal fluid circulation and by the cornea adapting slowly to its new environment.

Hill and Fatt[12] found that a securely fitted contact lens creates a rapid decrease in oxygen underneath itself. To demonstrate the need for oxygen underneath a contact lens, Smelser[13] added oxygen to the tear layer to create an oxygen bubble underneath the lens. He observed a gradual reduction in the size of the bubble as the oxygen was used by the cornea.

Clinical experience leads to recognition that the metabolic processes of the cornea must adapt to the new environment created by a corneal contact lens. Hence, the adaptive period for the new contact lens wearer may be considered to be the time required for the histochemical adjustment of the corneal metabolism to the vision aid. Although by weight a contact lens becomes a constant force against the corneal surface, there is little clinical evidence to suggest that it completely disturbs the orderly arrangement of the stroma fibrillae or affects the tissue fluid pressure of the cornea.

Adler[14] stated that the transparency of the cornea becomes temporarily impaired when abnormal pressures are applied to the cornea. He associated any loss of transparency not only with the imbibition of fluid but also with physical changes in the stroma, since the cloudiness disappears immediately when the pressure is decreased.

When a contact lens obstructs the cornea's access to oxygen, there is interference with the normal dehydration mechanism; the cornea becomes deturgesced, exhibiting increases in thickness and turbidity, and the lactic acid content increases. Coincident with the increase in lactic acid is an increase in the density, thickness, and water content of the cornea.

When a contact lens causes tears to be retained over the corneal surface, interference with tear evaporation at the surface occurs, and osmotic imbalance may result from either an increase in the salt content of the cornea or a decrease in the salt content of the tears. If we assume that the imbalance is caused by the former rather than the latter, we should be able to influence epithelial fluctuations by changing the contact lens design and thereby changing the composition of the tears.

STRUCTURE OF THE NORMAL CORNEA

Doggart[15] pointed out that biomicroscopy has proved that certain congenital abnormalities of the eye are more common than has generally been supposed. He added that although these abnormalities are found in as many as 50 percent of the people examined, many of them are trivial, require no treatment, and do not appreciably impair the function of the eye. The main concern of the patient and examiner is to know whether the condition is stationary or progressive. Doggart stated that limbal vessels, conjunctival vessels, and corneal nerves may vary in appearance in different patients so that a normal cornea may have several forms.

A preliminary survey of the cornea with the biomicroscope is made with sclerotic scatter, diffuse illumination, retro-illumination, indirect illumination, and the broad beam of direct illumination. The cornea is examined in depth for separate layers with the narrow beam of direct illumination (optical section).

Berens and Zuckerman[16] suggested that the practitioner first examine the cornea as a whole, noting its size, thickness, peripheral rings of opacification, and transition area at the limbus. Then the practitioner should observe the cornea in detail.

François and Rabaey[17] stated that the transparency or opacity of a tissue is determined by its structural frame and by the presence and concentration of certain substances. They used modern instrumentation and techniques—phase-contrast microscopy, historadiography, and electron microscope examinations—to describe corneal anatomy.

Epithelium

The epithelium consists of five cellular layers and is from 50 to 100 microns thick. The characteristics of the *basal cells* are as follows. The cells rest on Bowman's layer; are cylindrical, squat, or elongated; have an ellipsoid nucleous; and contain nucleic acid and deoxyribonucleic acid in the nucleus and ribonucleic acid in the cytoplasm.

The cells of the deepest row are dimpled, whereas the cells of the middle layer are irregularly polyhedral. The superficial cells are flat, retain their nucleus, and show no keratinization.

The human epithelium contains glycogen, which is a source of energy. Small granules, homogeneously spread, are found at the basal pole of the cell, which is difficult to see even with great magnification. François and Rabaey[18] believed that this pole indicated the existence of a strong bond between the polysaccharide and other tissue elements.

The corneal epithelium is rich in enzymes. The superficial layers contain less water than the other layers and have a chemical composition different from that of the other layers. The intercellular substance is a delicate cellular framework that delimits the cells of all parts and is found in the superficial and intermediary layers.

Phase contrast microscopy permits the examination of epithelial cells in vivo. It shows the cells as having a homogeneous nucleus with nucleoli and the cytoplasm as containing numerous granules that vary in arrangement in the cells of the different layers.

Electron microscope examination indicates that the epithelial cell wall is very irregular, especially in the basal and middle layers. The epithelial cells are surrounded by a membrane of irregular thickness. The cytoplasm is denser in the pseudopods and shows a network in which inclusions and granules are visible. The superficial cells show no vacuoles.

The epithelium can be examined with the biomicroscope, using diffuse illumination, direct illumination, indirect illumination, retro-illumination, and sclerotic scatter (not necessarily in this order). When the narrow beam of direct illumination is sharply focused on the anterior surface of the cornea, the anterior band is doubled; the second band to appear is very homogeneous and represents Bowman's layer. The space between the two corresponds to the epithelium, and purely epithelial changes are confined to this space.

With the narrow beam of direct illumination (optical section), the arc of the section always faces the direction of incident light and the epithelium is usually assumed to coincide with the anterior band. Doggart[19] described a variable epithelial edema on the limbal areas, which he believed was not necessarily an unfavorable sign. This condition, known as physiological bedewing of the epithelium (*bedewing* simply indicating a mild degree of edema that may be likened to the fine sprinkling of dewdrops on a lawn early in the morning), is observed with indirect illumination or retro-illumination. Apart from the peripheral bedewing, the normal epithelium shows no special characteristics when it is examined with the biomicroscope.

The basal membrane is a fine membrane that lies beneath the epithelial cells and supports them. Under the phase microscope it appears as a vividly red, thin, continuous margin.[20] It is thicker at the periphery, where its fibrillar structure is more evident. It contains no glycogen and is not chromotropic. The basal membrane contains plasmogen, which favors adhesion to the epithelial cells.

Bowman's Layer

Historadiographic examination shows Bowman's layer to be a fine, dense line underneath the basal cells and a less dense zone near the stroma. Electron microscopy has exposed a mosaic structure created by implantation of basal epithelial cells.

François and Rabaey[21] observed two zones: a dense band measuring 0.5 micron immediately below the epithelium and then a less dense band. The anterior surface is irregular and has crests that protrude among the basal cells. The posterior surface is not sharply circumscribed, and its fibers are continuous with the stroma fibers.

Jakus[22] considered Bowman's layer to be a modification of the stroma instead of a structureless membrane containing irregularly oriented fibrils similar to those within the lamellae of the stroma.

Seen through a biomicroscope, Bowman's layer is clearly defined by its thin white line. With the narrow beam of direct illumination in an optical section, it is observed to be between the epithelial layer and the stroma.

Stroma (Substantia Propia)

The stroma is the thickest layer of the cornea, occupying 90 percent of the cornea's entire thickness. With the biomicroscope it is seen to be nonvascular except at its extreme edge and to have an irregular, granular appearance and an iridescent glow when observed in optical section. The stroma is composed largely of water and collagen fibrils. The remaining solid material, comprising 0.15 percent of the total, contains lipids, water soluble extractives, some proteins insoluble in water, and the mucoid substance, which has been identified as mucopolysaccharide.[23]

The structure of the stroma is studied in the optical section or, if the beam is broad, on the lateral surface of the parallelepiped nearest the observer. Koby wrote:

> The stroma has a fairly regular marbled appearance which is due to the presence of small areas, *arachnoid corpuscles,* which are possibly identical with the fixed cells of the cornea. They appear to be connected both sagitally and frontally. The lamellar structure of the cornea seen in histological examination does not appear in the examination of the living eye and is probably an artifact caused by the reagents.[24]

Electron microscopy has shown that the sclera has thick collagen fibrils that vary in size, whereas the stromal fibrillae are delicate, identical and of uniform diameter. The corneal fibrallae are "dirty" in comparison with the fibrils of the sclera and usually stick together in a mass, as if they were enveloped by an amorphous substance, formed by the fibrillae, that covers the meshes. This amorphous substance is the mucoid.

The corneal mucoid appears to be responsible for the stromal property of rapid absorption of water from the environment. This property is important in the maintenance of corneal transparency. Transparency is normally assured as long as a certain equilibrium in hydration is maintained; increased water absorption immediately creates a loss of transparency. In a normal cornea, the compact mass of the fine fibrallae and mucoid creates an almost impossible barrier. A historadiographic examination shows the regular arrangement of the fibers parallel to the surface.

When François and Rabaey[25] examined the stroma after swelling, they found that the fibrillae were not thickened and that their structure was less serrated and slack. In their opinion, this finding supports the hypothesis that corneal swelling takes place exclusively in the interfibrillar mucoid.

Duke-Elder[26] stated that in inflammatory conditions the cornea thickens and the stroma suffers a loss of transparency and appears to be milky white. Infiltrations and thickenings—localized, diffuse, or disciform—can be delineated, and fine opacities can be observed.

Descemet's Membrane

Descemet's membrane has a thickness of 6 microns and, on routine histological or phase contrast microscopy, appears to have no structure. Baud and Balavoine[27] described Descemet's membrane as consisting of superimposed lamellae, parallel with the surface. Electron microscope examination shows a granulated, undulated structure with surface irregularities measuring 0.05 to 0.1 microns.

In a biomicroscope optical section, Descemet's membrane appears as a thin, narrow grey line immediately posterior to the stroma. In pathological conditions it is frequently folded, indicating the involvement of the deep layers after either inflammation or trauma; the folding (wavy appearance) usually occurs in conditions of hypotony. This layer can separate itself from the stroma or reduplicate itself after surgery.

Endothelium

Phase contrast microscopy of the corneal endothelium shows it to be a single layer of flat cells suspended in aqueous humor. This thin sheet of predominantly hexagonal cells approximately 20 microns in diameter and 5 microns deep shows morphological evidence of considerable metabolic activity.[28] Descemet's membrane is the basement membrane for the endothelium. The posterior border of the cells is free and in direct contact with the aqueous humor. Endothelial cells have a large oval or flat nucleus that is centrally located. The cytoplasm shows a large number of granulations varying in volume, which indicates intensive cellular activity.

Tripathi[29] described the endothelium as being rich in intracellular organelles (for example, numerous mitochondria, well-developed Golgi apparatus, endoplasmic reticulum, ribosomes, and glycogen granules), which indicate its active metabolic state. The endothelium is the more important barrier to water.

After investigations with the electron micrograph, Jakus[30] reported that the endothelial cytoplasm comprises numerous inclusions and infolded membranes. François and Rabaey,[31] commenting that these osmophilic infolded membranes, or B-cytomembranes, are present where water transport is very active, concluded that these cells are actively involved in the transfer of water between the anterior chamber and the cornea.

A bicarbonate dependent sodium pump operates across the endothelium, translocating material from the stroma back into the aqueous humor. This pump-leak mechanism controls the corneal water relationships and helps keep the cornea transparent.[32]

The endothelium is not visible with biomicroscopic optical section. However, small sections can be observed in the zone of specular reflection. Doggart[33] described the endothelial cells as having well-defined outlines that appear to be dark, with their shape usually hexagonal, sometimes pentagonal, and occasionally square and the cell layer having a honeycombed appearance. According to Doggart, the endothelium near the limbus looks like it is interrupted by a series of punched out holes. The holes are caused by localized, backward extensions of Descemet's membrane, named Hassal-Henle warts. They are most often found in adults and the elderly. Whereas the original purpose of endothelial examination was to assess the suitability of the donor cornea and posterior corneal damage following cataract surgery and intraocular lens implants, biomicroscopic examination of the corneal endothelium is becoming more significant to contact lens practitioners.[34]

The relationship between endothelial cells and contact lens wear was given significance by Zantos and Holden,[35] who described changes in the endothelial mosaic following soft contact lens wear. Black areas called *endothelial blebs* appear between adjacent cells within 10 minutes after soft contact lenses are inserted. However, there is a gradual decrease in the disturbance with continued wearing of the lenses. The endothelial mosaic returns to normal within an hour after lens removal.

Limbal Area

Koby[36] described the limbal area as being less well defined when it is observed with a biomicroscope than when it is observed with the naked eye. Whitish radial fibrous tracts arising from the sclera encroach on the cornea and occupy a peripheral zone (palisade zone). The vessels form a fine, freely anastomosing network at the limbus; in the palisade zone the vessels have a radial distribution and their fine anastomoses extend in fairly regular arcades to the edge of the zone.

With the biomicroscopic techniques of indirect illumination and retro-illumination, the lamp being placed at a severely acute angle (65° to 80°), physiological edema of the cornea is found at the extreme peripheral corneal areas. The edema can be observed with both low and high magnification. Since the limbal palisades can be seen with high magnification, the extent and characteristics of the limbal vessels should be studied so that in contact lens practice, a prefitting corneal examination of their appearance can be recorded for future reference.

With diffuse illumination one can observe how scleral vessels extend to the limbus and encroach on the outer corneal peripheral areas. In some patients the limbal palisades are well defined; in others the areas of physiological edema may obscure limbal definition so that, with broad beam diffuse or direct illumination, one can observe a 1 mm to 2 mm wide grey area between the sclera and cornea.

When using biomicroscopy to examine the limbus, one can expect to find wide variations; these variations are normal for individual patients. For contact lens practice, it is important to record the appearance of limbal palisades and their corneal extension.

Corneal Nerve Filaments

In 1830, Schlemm first described corneal nerves. In 1837, Bochdaalek confirmed Schlemm's report that the corneal nerves originate in the ciliary nerves and consist of deep and superficial branches that terminate on the corneal surface.[37]

The corneal nerves form an annular plexus at the limbus, usually in the posterior two-thirds, so that the larger nerve fibers are in the deeper layers and the finer filaments are nearer the anterior surface. Nerve filaments look like strands of silk. The corneal nerves pass into the stroma in the deeper layers, lose their myelin sheaths within the first millimeter, and branch dichotomously (with an angle of 30° to 60° between themselves), the branches usually having unequal lengths. (Trichotomous branching and further branch subdivisions are sometimes seen.) The branches then form networks at three levels: one within the stroma, one under Bowman's layer, and one within the epithelium. There are no specialized end organs. Rodger, who studied the so-called free nerve endings in the epithelium, found that these endings were not within the epithelial cells but on and between them and that, in some instances, they reached the surface to form long arcades immediately below the outermost layer of the stratified squamous epithelium.[38]

Corneal nerves are best seen with an optical section and the incident light at a wide angle (45° to 70°). Their course can be examined when the light beam is focused on them, although the surrounding areas are out of focus. Berliner[39] stated that the number of corneal nerves may be between 30 and 50.

In the limbal areas, the corneal nerves may enter the cornea in radial directions so that they resemble spearlike projections under indirect illumination. The courses of corneal nerves can be followed better with high magnification. Although it is rather easy to observe corneal nerves that are near the anterior part of the cornea, the nerves appear to lose their definition and end abruptly when their course is traced to the deeper corneal layers, where they terminate.

The corneal nerves become more visible when inflammatory corneal lesions are present. These lesions may cause fine, sleevelike infiltrates to surround the nerves. However, a loss of normal corneal transparency also occurs, interfering with the increased visibility.[40]

Corneal Sensitivity

A distinction can be made between *corneal sensibility* and *corneal sensitivity*. The former describes the cornea's ability to feel or perceive a stimulus at its surface; the latter describes the cornea's ability to transmit a sensation and respond to it.

The cornea is known to have free nerve endings on its surface. Touch receptors are present, but heat receptors are not. The cornea has a highly developed sensitivity for superficial pain, although large variations in individual response are found. A decrease in corneal sensitivity from the central areas to the periphery is noticed, with highest sensitivity found in a circular zone immediately surrounding the center of the cornea. Pain sensitivity corresponds to the distribution of nerves, since there is a rich supply of free nerve endings in the central corneal areas. Pain caused by corneal irritation is felt as a foreign body sensation. Although receptors for heat and for pain caused by heat are absent, receptors for touch, pressure, and general pain do exist, their response depending on the intensity of the stimulus. Cold receptors lie at a deeper level than the free nerve endings and give rise to painful sensations. Also, the sensation of cold is more resistant to anesthesia than is the sense of pain. Even without heat receptors, pain stimuli can induce a subjective feeling of heat. Corneal stimuli are conducted to the central nervous system by the ophthalmic division of the fifth cranial nerve.

Photophobia—pain induced by exposure to light—is believed to be caused by referred pain, which results from the close association of the fifth nerve and the optic nerve. This relationship is demonstrated when the condition is relieved by topical anesthesia.

According to Thomas,[41] the water content of the epithelium apparently is regulated by the nerves. Thomas reported that the amount of water in the epithelial cells was increased after irritation of the trigeminal nerve, so that after section of the trigeminal nerve the epithelium became edematous and islands of cells were desquamated, leaving pits in the corneal surface.

Various methods used to test corneal sensitivity rely on adjustable nylon threads, hairs, and so on for touching the cornea in different areas. Mandell[42] commented that testing with a battery of hairs of different values is impractical since the hairs can change with the moisture of the surrounding atmosphere. The length and bend of the filaments are altered while the pressure application is continued until there is a threshold of sensation. These devices, known as corneal aesthesiometers, corneal sensibilometers, and so on have been introduced by Boberg-Ans[43] and Schirmer and Mellor.[44] Their use in contact lens practice has been described by Strughold[45] and others.

A Cochet and Bonnet aesthesiometer can be used for routine measurements of corneal sensation. It tests the sensitivity of the upper lid in the center of the tarsal conjunctiva, near the lid margin on its conjunctival surface, and on the peripheral corneal areas to the edge of the pupils both before and after adaptation to a daily contact lens wearing schedule.

Schirmer,[46] Koetting,[47] and Kraar and Cummings[48] have reported on the use of an aesthesiometer to measure corneal sensitivity prior to the fitting of contact lenses. Significant differences in corneal sensitivity can be found among control groups tested with an aesthesiometer. Schirmer[49] reported that people with lower sensitivities adjust better to contact lenses. However, these conclusions have not been correlated with generally accepted contact lens fitting procedures. Although some patients exhibit a more sensitive reaction to contact lenses than do others, a poor initial response to contact lenses may have a psychological basis.

Stating that wide fluctuations in corneal sensitivity exist among patients, Bier[50] considered it preferable to make individual tests for corneal sensitivity prior to fitting contact lenses. Success in wearing contact lenses depends on a multitude of factors, and the results of corneal sensitivity studies are far from conclusive. Information about corneal sensitivity may in the future prove to be valuable in the prognosis of successful wearing of contact lenses; but on the basis of present knowledge, corneal hypersensitivity cannot be considered a definite contraindication to the fitting of contact lenses. In fact, a contact lens patient with reduced corneal sensitivity may need closer observation than the normal patient does to make certain that abrasions undetected by the patient do not occur.

Bier[51] and Dixon[52] have reported that the sensitivity to touch of the cornea decreases in patients who habitually wear contact lenses. Corneal sensitivity decreases after the age of 45; a person 60 years old has about half the sensitivity of a person under 20. Millidot[53] has reported a 50 percent reduction in sensitivity by 70 years of age. He also has found that sensitivity is greatest in blue-eyed individuals. Sensitivity is also reduced by surgical interference and old scars. However, contact lens wearers regain corneal sensitivity shortly after removing the lenses; recovery may vary among all-day wearers.

The patient who wears contact lenses for the first time is immediately aware of a foreign body sensation, with lacrimation and epiphora. As wearing time is built up, the patient adapts to the lenses and no longer feels this sensation. Corneal and lid sensitivity is gradually reduced as adaptation to contact lens wear increases. Dixon[54] commented that this is consistent with the findings of Adrian and Zotterman, who reported that a steady stimulus caused a rapid decline in the rhythm of a sensory nerve impulse and who postulated that this decline might be due to a decrease in the excitability of the end organs, to a gradual increase in their refractory period, or both.

The reduction in corneal sensitivity that may cause contact lens wearers to be unaware of corneal involvement during lens wear emphasizes the need for periodic examinations with the biomicroscope. Aphakic patients, as well as others who have reduced corneal sensitivity, may experience minor superficial epithelial abrasions when inserting contact lenses and be unaware of them.

Sensitivity decreases among hard lens wearers but returns to normal several hours after the lens is removed; recovery is slow. There is no reduction in corneal thickness. As for sensitivity loss caused by contact lens wear, Millidot[55] found a 45 percent reduction caused by soft lenses and a 110 percent reduction caused by hard lenses.

CORNEAL TEMPERATURES

Corneal temperatures are relatively low in comparison to those of the body or other parts of the eye. The lowest temperature is at the corneal apex (92° F). Although the limbus is normally warmer because of its greater vascularity, the highest temperature is found beneath the upper lid.[56]

It is doubtful that temperature receptors are present in the cornea; however, it was found that in rabbits fitted with scleral and corneal lenses the corneal temperature increased initially 6° F, decreased after 2 or 3 minutes of lens wear, and became stabilized at approximately the temperature found during the examination, before fitting. Yet the temperature increased during eye closure (blink or forced blink) while the animals wore the contact lens, and this result was found to be essentially duplicated in humans fitted with scleral lenses.[57]

Although authorities agree that there are no corneal heat receptors, contact lens patients report subjective symptoms of burning and stinging that appear to be related to the presence of temperature receptors. According to Hill and Fatt,[58] contact lens wear has little effect on corneal temperature when the eyelids are open and the patient's gaze is in the primary position. The temperature apparently increases when the patient blinks or when fixation changes reduce the vertical dimensions of the palpebral fissure. It would seem, therefore, that the fitting of corneal lenses within the palpebral fissure, resulting in their minimum movement or displacement in blinking, may actually provide the most compatible physiological lens-cornea relationship.

CORNEAL EPITHELIAL TURNOVER

In early studies, the corneal epithelium was described as being a relatively thin tissue six to eight cells deep of stratified squamous epithelium, the deepest cells being elongated or columnar, the middle cells polyhedral, and the superficial cells somewhat flattened. It was assumed that each layer undergoes cell regeneration separately.[59]

In 1960, Hanna and O'Brien[60] used tritium labeled thymidine as a cell marker. The marker was incorporated into the cell nucleus during the premitotic phase, becoming stable during the remainder of the cell's existence and permitting study of the proliferation and subsequent function of the epithelial cells of the cornea. Thymidine was injected into the anterior chamber of rats' eyes, and the eyes were enucleated at hourly intervals to be studied for the extent of labeling. The amount of tritium labeled thymidine incorporated into the cells diminished in about 4 hours, and the degree of labeling became lighter. It was thus possible to distinguish between recently labeled cells and associated migration. The basal cells migrated forward and reached the superficial layers in an average of 3 days. Although some of the cells sloughed off within 3 days, a complete turnover of cells occurred within 7 days. This proliferating activity, plus limiting dimensions of the corneal epithelium layer thickness, caused the cell structure to become more compressed as the cells approached the outer layers of the cornea.

Contact lens wear requires that the cornea support a constant mass remaining in position (14 to 16 hours average for all-day wearers) while new basal cells are formed in this environment. However, no report has yet described how this factor influences changes in the basal cell structure of the corneal epithelium over a period of time.

CORNEAL VASCULARIZATION

A symptom of an inflammatory disturbance, corneal vascularization occurs when the cornea loses its tissue compactness. Although the condition is readily cured and the cornea appears to be normal, the vessel walls never disappear.

The cornea is normally avascular and derives its nutrition from the pericorneal vessels. In inflammatory conditions, the cornea obtains an additional blood supply from pericorneal congestion or injection of the normal limbal vessels and from the formation of new vessels (neoformations), which vascularize the cornea.

Dixon[61] described the development of corneal vascularization among animals fitted experimentally with scleral contact lenses. Lauber,[62] Strebel,[63] Delgado,[64] and others reported corneal vascularization induced in human subjects by contact lenses. All observers reported that after wearing was discontinued the blood disappeared from the vessels.

Ashton[65] showed that a zone of corneal swelling extending to the limbus is essential to the development of vascularization. Cogan and Kinsey[66] suggested that corneal edema is an important factor if it is prolonged and if it involves an area near the limbal vessels. A limbal obstruction capable of reducing corneal tissue compactness can cause corneal edema and vascularization.

In corneal lens patients, vascularization is usually caused by overfilling of the limbal vessels. Occasionally, the vessels proliferate a short distance into the clear cornea.

The cornea does not become vascularized when a contact lens induces epithelial trauma because the cornea does not lose its tissue compactness. However, neglect and poor clinical management of a contact lens fit may cause loss in compactness, with resultant stromal edema and vascularization. Biomicroscope photography may be used to record the appearance of limbal vessels prior to the fitting of contact lenses and throughout all aftercare periods.

A distinction should be made between the corneal vascularization that occurs in general pathological conditions (that is, the presence of new vessels filled with blood in the stroma) and the appearance of new vessels filled with blood on the superficial epithelial surfaces in the limbal areas in contact lens wearers. Johnson and Erkhardt[67] explained the proliferation of capillaries from the limbus into the cornea as an attempt by the latter to bring oxygen to its cells in response to corneal asphyxia. We might question the continued use of the term *corneal vascularization* to describe the condition in which limbal vessels overfill and proliferate for short distances into the clear peripheral corneal areas of some contact lens wearers. Instead, we might consider using the term *limbal vessel proliferation* for the purpose of clarity and distinctive reference. Since a variable degree of physiological edema and tissue compactness exists in the limbal (outer peripheral) corneal areas, we may expect to find a high incidence of limbal vascular changes, including trauma and limbal vessel proliferations, when contact lens peripheral dimensions and the position of the lens on the cornea cause asphyxia.

COMMENTARY

Contact lenses are foreign bodies; they may produce corneal physio-logical changes by causing trauma, by altering corneal metabolism, and by changing the levels of sensation and oxygen tension. These possibilities are eliminated when contact lens design variables are compatible with all of the factors related to the maintenance of corneal transparency.

Only a small amount of the cornea is exposed to atmospheric oxygen when it is covered with a contact lens; the amount of exposure is related to the overall lens size and the lid opening. Contact lens wear so reduces the amount of atmospheric oxygen supplied to the cornea that oxygen tension behind a contact lens is below that of atmospheric partial pressure (155 mm Hg) and the amount of dissolved oxygen in the cornea decreases.[68] Although the deeper layers of the corneal epithelium have a lower oxygen tension and the superficial epithelial layers use almost all of the available oxygen for their aerobic metabolism, the deeper epithelial layers can obtain oxygen by diffusion from the uncovered areas or from the aqueous humor when the oxygen tension is low at the epithelial side (as when the lids are closed). The epithelium may experience various degrees of oxygen deprivation during contact lens wear; however, sustained damage may be precluded by the rapid rate of epithelial regeneration.

The cornea adapts to oxygen deprivation by some unknown mechanism or by use of an alternate pathway (for example, the reduction branch of the glycolytic pathway) that requires less oxygen from the atmosphere to maintain the metabolic processes responsible for corneal transparency.[69] When the lens design is improper or the wearing time is incompatible with the adaptation rate, pathological conditions such as edema, abrasions, pain, and vascularization result. It has been suggested that during wearing periods, when the amount of dissolved oxygen in the cornea decreases, prolonged oxygen tension changes may affect corneal contour.[70] After contact lens removal, the cornea readapts to the increased oxygen supply and returns to prewear levels of metabolic function.

NOTES

1. J. François and M. Rabaey, "The Anatomy of the Cornea," in *The Transparency of the Cornea,* ed. S. Duke-Elder and E. S. Perkins (Oxford, England: Blackwell Scientific Publications, 1960).

2. D. M. Maurice, *The Cornea and Sclera,* vol. 1 of *In the Eye,* ed. H. Davson (New York: Academic Press, 1962).

3. H. Davson, *The Physiology of the Eye,* 2d ed. (Boston: Little, Brown, 1963).

4. Ibid.

5. Ibid.; G. K. Smelser and V. I. Ozanics, "Importance of Atmospheric Oxygen for Maintenance of the Optical Properties of the Human Cornea," *Science* 115 (February 1, 1952): 140.

6. D. G. Cogan and V. E. Kinsey, "Cornea: Physiological Aspects," *Archives of Ophthalmology* 28 (October 1942): 661–669.

7. D. M. Maurice, "The Permeability of the Cornea," in Duke-Elder and Perkins, *Transparency of the Cornea.*

8. F. H. Adler, *Physiology of the Eye: Clinical Application,* 3d ed. (St. Louis: C. V. Mosby, 1959).

9. N. Ashton, "Corneal Vascularization," in Duke-Elder and Perkins, *Transparency of the Cornea.*

10. G. K. Smelser and D. K. Chen, "Physiological Changes in Cornea Induced by Contact Lenses," *Archives of Ophthalmology* 53 (March 1955): 676–679.

11. J. Hirano, "Histological Studies on the Corneal Changes Induced by Corneal Contact Lenses," *Japanese Journal of Ophthalmology* 3 (January–March 1959): 1–8.

12. R. M. Hill and I. Fatt, "Oxygen Measurements under a Contact Lens," *American Journal of Optometry* 41 (June 1964): 382–387.

13. G. L. Smelser, "Relation of Factors Involved in Maintenance of Optical Properties of Cornea to Contact Lens Wear," *Archives of Ophthalmology* 47 (March 1952): 328–343.

14. Adler, *Physiology of the Eye.*

15. J. H. Doggart, *Ocular Signs in Slit-Lamp Microscopy* (St. Louis: C. V. Mosby, 1949).

16. C. Berens and J. Zuckerman, *Diagnostic Examination of the Eye* (Philadelphia: Lippincott, 1946).

17. François and Rabaey, "Anatomy of the Cornea."

18. Ibid.

19. Doggart, *Ocular Signs in Slit-Lamp Microscopy.*

20. A. J. La Tessa et al., "Histochemistry of Basement Membrane of Cornea," *American Journal of Ophthalmology* 38 (August 1954): 171–177; L. Calmettes et al., "Etude histologique et histochemique de l'epithelium anterieur de la cornée et de ses basales," *Archives of Ophthalmology* 16 (July–August 1956): 481–506.

21. François and Rabaey, "Anatomy of the Cornea."

22. M. A. Jakus, *Ocular Fine Structure: Selected Electron Micrographs* (Boston: Little, Brown, 1964).

23. G. I. Thomas, *The Cornea* (Springfield, Ill.: Charles C. Thomas, 1955).

24. F. E. Koby, *Slit-Lamp Microscopy of the Living Eye,* trans, C. Goulden and C. L. Harris (Philadelphia: P. Blakiston's Sons, 1930), p. 36.

25. François and Rabaey, "Anatomy of the Cornea."

26. S. Duke-Elder, ed., *System of Ophthalmology,* vol. 7 (St. Louis: C. V. Mosby, 1962).

27. C. A. Baud and C. Balavoine, "L'ultrastructure de la membrane de Descemet et de ses derives pathologiques (stries hyalines)," *Ophthalmologica (Basel)* 126 (November 1953): 390–394.

28. R. C. Tripathi, "Applied Physiology and Anatomy," in *Contact Lens Practice,* ed. M. Ruben (New York: Macmillan, 1975), pp. 24–55.

29. Ibid.

30. M. A. Jakus, "Studies on the Cornea: II. The Fine Structure of Descemet's Membrane," *Journal of Biophysical Cytology* 2 (July 1956): 25.

31. François and Rabaey, "Anatomy of the Cornea."

32. S. T. Parrish, "The Corneal Endothelium: A Review of Its Clinical Observation and Implications in Contact Lens Practice," *Journal of the British Contact Lens Association* 4 (January 1981): 10–16.

33. Doggart, *Ocular Signs in Slit-Lamp Microscopy.*

34. Parrish, "Corneal Endothelium."

35. S. Zantos and B. Holden, "High Magnification Examination and Photography with the Slit-Lamp," in *Clinical Slit-Lamp Biomicroscopy,* ed. R. H. Brandreth (San Leandro, Calif.: Blaco Printers, 1978), pp. 329–342.

36. Koby, *Slit-Lamp Microscopy of the Living Eye.*

37. Thomas, *Cornea.*

38. Ibid.

39. M. L. Berliner, *Biomicroscopy of the Eye* (London: Hamish Hamilton Medical Books, 1949).

40. Ibid.

41. Thomas, *Cornea.*

42. R. B. Mandell, *Contact Lens Practice: Basic and Advanced* (Springfield, Ill.: Charles C. Thomas, 1965).

43. J. Boberg-Ans, "Experience in Clinical Examination of Corneal Sensitivity: Corneal Sensitivity and Nasolacrimal Reflex after Retrobulbular Anaesthesia," *British Journal of Ophthalmology* 39 (December 1955): 705–726.

44. K. E. Schirmer and L. D. Mellor, "Corneal Sensitivity after Cataract Extraction," *Archives of Ophthalmology* 65 (March 1961): 433–436.

45. H. Strughold, "The Sensitivity of Cornea and Conjunctiva of the Human Eye and the Use of Contact Lenses," *American Journal of Optometry* 30 (December 1953): 625–630.

46. K. E. Schirmer, "Corneal Sensitivity and Contact Lenses," *British Journal of Ophthalmology* 47 (August 1963): 493–495.

47. R. A. Koetting, "Useful Auxilliary Tests in Contact Lens Examination," *American Optometric Association Journal* 36 (August 1965): 439–442.

48. R. S. Kraar and C. M. Cummings, "Lacrimation, Corneal Sensitivity and Corneal Abrasive Resistance in Contact Lens Wearability," *Optometric Weekly,* November 18, 1965, pp. 25–32.

49. Schirmer, "Corneal Sensitivity and Contact Lenses."

50. N. Bier, "The Cornea's Reaction to Contact Lenses" (paper delivered at the New England Council of Optometrists Meeting, Boston, Mass., March 13–16, 1966).

51. N. Bier, *Contact Lens Routine and Practice* (London: Butterworths Scientific Publishers, 1957).

52. J. M. Dixon, "Ocular Changes Due to Contact Lenses," *American Journal of Ophthalmology* 58 (September 1964): 424–443.

53. M. Millidot, "Corneal Sensitivity and Contact Lenses" (paper delivered at the Eighth National Research Symposium on Contact Lenses, sponsored by Bausch & Lomb, Boston, Mass., August 1981).

54. Dixon, "Ocular Changes Due to Contact Lenses."

55. M. Millidot, *Acta Ophthalmologica* 54 (1976): 721.

56. Mandell, *Contact Lens Practice.*

57. R. M. Hill and A. J. Leighton, "Physiological Time Courses Associated with Contact Lenses—Temperature: I. Animal Time Courses with Scleral Lenses," *American Journal of Optometry* 40 (August 1963): 427–438; R. M. Hill and A. J. Leighton, "Physiological Time Courses Associated with Contact Lenses—Temperature: II. Animal Time Courses with Corneal Lenses," *American Journal of Optometry* 41 (January 1964): 3–9; R. M. Hill and A. J. Leighton, "Temperature Changes of Human Cornea and Tears under Contact Lenses: I. The Relaxed Open Eye and the Natural and Forced Closed Eye Conditions," *American Journal of Optometry* 42 (January 1965): 9–16; R. M. Hill and A. J. Leighton, "Temperature Changes of Human Cornea and Tears under Contact Lenses: II. Effects of Intermediate Lid Apertures and Gaze," *American Journal of Optometry* 42 (February 1965): 71–77.

58. Hill and Fatt, "Oxygen Measurements."

59. H. E. Jordan, *The Textbook of Histology* (New York: Appleton-Century-Crofts, 1937).

60. C. Hanna and J. E. O'Brien, "All Production and Migration in the Epithelial Layer of the Cornea," *Archives of Ophthalmology* 64 (1960): 536–591.

61. Dixon, "Ocular Changes."

62. H. Lauber in discussion on A. Deutsch, "Praktische Durchfuhrung von Myopie-korrektion mit Kontaktglasern," *Klinische Monatsblatter fur Augen-heilkunde (Stuttgart)* 82 (1929): 535.

63. J. Strebel, "Objective Proof for the Orthopedic Effect of Contact Lenses on Keratoconus," *Klinische Monatsblatter fur Augenheilkunde (Stuttgart)* 99 (July 1937): 30–35.

64. Dixon, "Ocular Changes."

65. Ashton, "Corneal Vascularization."

66. Cogan and Kinsey, "Cornea: Physiological Aspects."

67. L. V. Johnson and R. E. Erkhardt, "Rosacea Keratitis and Conditions with Vascularization of the Cornea Treated with Riboflavin," *Archives of Ophthalmology* 23 (1940): 902.

68. M. Ruben, "Recent Developments in Contact Lens Practice," *Contact Lens Journal* 1 (October 1967): 5–10.

69. R. L. Farris, G. H. Takahashi, and A. Donn, "Corneal Oxygen Flux in Contact Lens Wearers," in *Corneal and Scleral Lenses,* ed. L. J. Girard (St. Louis: C. V. Mosby, 1967).

70. Ruben, *Recent Developments.*

Chapter 4

Examination Technique

In contact lens practice, the low power objective of the biomicroscope is used more often than the high power objectives for the initial examination procedures because it has a greater depth of focus and a wider field of vision. High power objectives are used to study the cornea and any irregularities in detail. The slit can be adjusted from a hairline to a wide, open, circular aperture. The design of the joy stick biomicroscope makes it possible for one hand to operate the stage and focus the microscope while the other hand controls the angle and width of the incident light.

Biomicroscopy should not replace any system that is used for either gross examination of the eye or examination of the contact lens fit. A conventional lamp that is used for black light fluorescein examination of the eye should not be discarded. A blue filter is usually part of the biomicroscope's equipment. A fluorescein and black light examination is used to assess the characteristics of the contact lens fit for clearance and bearing areas; the illumination and magnification of a biomicroscope can be used for examining contact lens fit in greater detail.

THE VARIANT OF CORNEAL APPEARANCE

Koby[1] presented a fascinating discussion of the phenomena of light reflection by the ocular media. He stated that the ocular media are composed of several *zones of discontinuity*—optical surfaces where the index of refraction suddenly changes. A luminous beam striking such a zone provokes certain optical phenomena, of which reflection is important to biomicroscopy; the others are refraction, polarization, diffraction, and fluorescence. One part of the rays is reflected according to the laws of *regular reflection,* the reflected rays being contained in the same plane as the incident rays and their respective angles being equal.

The quantity of reflected light in biomicroscopy depends chiefly on (1) differences of indices of refraction of the media considered, (2) the degree of polish of the reflecting surface, and (3) the size of the angle of incidence. Reflected light regularly produces an image of the luminous source at the point of convergence of the rays (real image) or of prolongation of the rays (virtual image); the observer in the path of regularly reflected rays receives the specular reflection of the surface (its reflex).

One part of the incident light is reflected in a diffuse, irregular fashion; this phenomenon, noticed on the surface of all bodies, makes the bodies visible. Thus biomicroscopy produces the phenomenon of light in the ocular media. The diffuse reflection that occurs at each zone of discontinuity makes it possible to distinguish among the various corneal layers.

The cornea has a complex, heterogeneous cellular structure. (The structure of glass is homogeneous.) The internal dispersion of light caused by the heterogeneity of semitransparent tissues is known as *relucency*. When the cornea is examined with the biomicroscope, it is seen to vary in appearance according to the type of illumination used. When it is examined with diffuse illumination, it appears to be transparent. When the illumination is direct, an opalescent block of light is formed and the optical effects of the corneal anatomy observed depend on the transparency of the tissues traversed.

EXAMINATION PROCEDURE

The following examination procedure should be used in all instances:

1. Lower the room illumination and adjust the instrument to make the patient comfortable.
2. Instruct the patient to place his or her chin on the chinrest and forehead against the headrest while the instrument is adjusted to the proper height.
3. Turn on the instrument and, if a fixation light is used, close the slit diaphragm and instruct the patient to gaze toward the fixation light. If such a light is not used, instruct the patient to gaze toward your right ear when the right eye is to be examined and toward your left ear when the left eye is to be examined.

ILLUMINATION METHODS

One does not selectively use each illumination method in turn, since, as Doggart noted, "in actual practice the methods of illumination overlap and swiftly alternate with each other."[2] Clinical procedures for biomicroscope corneal examination are determined empirically. The order of their use is determined by the individual examiner. The principal illumination methods are sclerotic scatter, diffuse illumination, direct illumination, transillumination or retro-illumination, indirect illumination, specular reflection, and oscillation.

The first six of the seven illumination methods are considered the principal ones (although they are not necessarily in their order of importance here). The seventh, oscillation, serves an auxiliary function. All seven methods are available for biomicroscope examination of the anterior segment of the globe, and the efficiency of the instrument in the finer points of diagnosis is related to the selection, application, and control of the proper method.

The cornea is observed in optical section according to its histology. The examination should begin with the epithelium and continue with Bowman's layer, the stroma, Descemet's membrane, and the endothelium. Although, as mentioned, the methods for complete corneal examination are related, there is no established procedure. Consequently, the illumination methods will be described in their listed order for the purpose of suggesting a clinical procedure sequence—the order of presentation not indicating the importance. Here the indirect forms of illumination will be elected for the initial corneal survey (since light is not focused directly on the cornea, patients will be more comfortable at the start); the examination will be continued with the direct forms.

Sclerotic Scatter

A special variety of indirect illumination is sclerotic scatter. The light is out of focus on the cornea, and the microscope is focused on the cornea (see Figure 4–1). An intense beam of light is directed to the sclera near the temporal limbus; the light crisscrosses the limiting membranes of the cornea and illuminates the circumcorneal region to create a *circumcorneal halo,* which appears as an orange-colored glow around the cornea. Light is reflected backward and forward between the two limiting surfaces of the cornea and is scattered centrifugally around the cornea. Sclerotic scatter exposes areas where the cornea is not transparent.

The procedure is as follows:

1. Narrow the light beam and direct it to the temporal-limbal area of the cornea. If there is a prism at the top of the lamp, it can be rotated to direct the light.
2. Move the lamp and microscope toward the patient's eye until the light is directed to the proper area.

The lamp is usually at an angle of 30° to 60° on the temporal side of the patient's eye, and the examiner may have to change the angle of incident light and coordinate this action with focusing the microscope on the cornea until the circumcorneal halo is formed. The adjacent area of the cornea is lit because of its own relucency;

Figure 4–1. Sclerotic scatter. Courtesy of Charles Erickson.

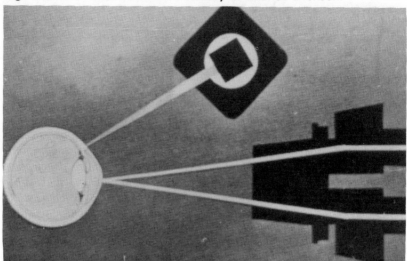

a similar glow is observed at other corneal peripheral areas, particularly the side opposite, as the circumcorneal halo is formed.

Sclerotic scatter permits observation of the following:

1. *Corneal staining when sodium fluorescein is used.* Irregularities appear as shadows, which can be studied in greater detail with other types of illumination.
2. *Contact lens scratches.* Surface scratches and irregularities of the lenses are exposed. They require detailed study with other types of illumination.
3. *Quality of lacrimal flow when contact lenses are worn.* The tears are normally transparent, and lacrimal flow is observed only when reference materials, such as lacrimal debris and various particles, are present beneath the lens.
4. *Interference with corneal metabolism.* Because there may be an improper lens-cornea relationship, observations may include epithelial disturbances such as punctuate, stippling, epithelial edema, irregular edematous lines, epithelial dimpling, and any loss of continuity of the epithelial surface (see Figure 4–2).
5. *Central corneal clouding.* This circular, disclike edematous formation in the central corneal area (generally over the pupil) can be induced by oxygen deprivation, focalized corneal bearing, or both when firm corneal lenses are fitted. It is easily exposed when the biomicroscope has a prism at the top of the lamp that can be rotated so that the incident light to the

Figure 4–2. Sclerotic scatter, high magnification. The incident light, from the examiner's left, creates a circumcorneal halo around the limbal-scleral junction to the examiner's right. Scattered stained corneal punctates are observed in shadow, although some of the light is reflected from the punctates in the lower left part of the cornea. (This is a biophotograph of a demonstration eye used for teaching.)

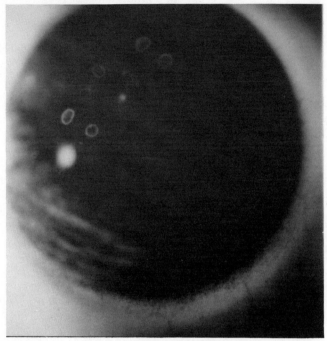

cornea is at a very oblique angle. It is difficult to observe this condition without the aid of the prism, although it is sometimes possible to detect the gray-white cloudy appearance of the edematous area macroscopically or through the instrument by moving the lamp housing arm laterally (see Figure 4–3).

6. *Lens position for hydrogel or silicone elastomer contact lenses.* Sclerotic scatter is used to observe the lens position for orientation over the cornea and its movement characteristics on blinking. It also exposes the presence of deposits on the anterior surface of the lens, although not to the degree possible with direct illumination or retro-illumination.

Diffuse Illumination
Out-of-focus incident light is directed to the cornea and provides a general picture of the anterior corneal surface with diffuse illumination (see Figure 4–4). The iris and limbal areas are illuminated, and obvious corneal changes are revealed.

Figure 4–3. Sclerotic scatter, high magnification, showing corneal edema in the apical area over the pupil (also called central corneal clouding or disc edema). Incident light scattered through the cornea exposes a central corneal edematous area. (This is a biophotograph of a demonstration eye used for teaching.)

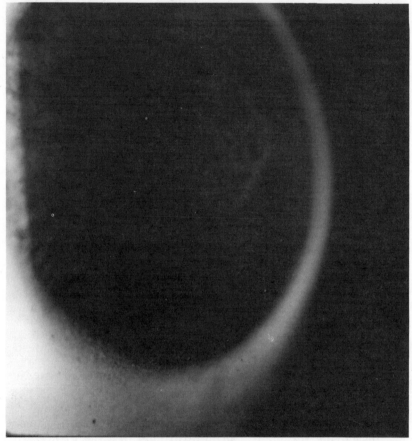

When this type of illumination is used to observe the fit of a firm corneal lens, tinting the tears with sodium fluorescein and using a blue filter will enhance the diagnostic procedure. The procedure itself is as follows:

1. Make the beam 2 mm wide or wider.
2. Direct incident light to the eye at oblique angles (30° to 50°).
3. Move the microscope toward the patient's eye and focus on the area to be observed.

The light illuminates the entire corneal surface, although it is not in focus.

Figure 4–4. Diffuse illumination. Courtesy of Charles Erickson.

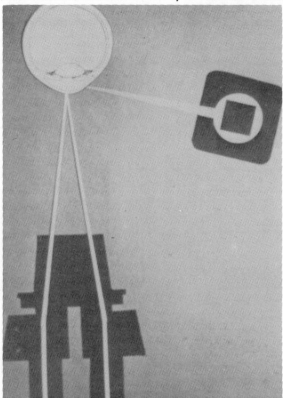

Diffuse illumination permits the observation of the cornea, sclera, lids, and conjunctiva. It also permits the study of contact lens surface characteristics, lacrimal flow characteristics indicated by the movement of lacrimal debris and particles beneath the corneal lens, and aspects of contact lens fit, including scleral encroachment, limbal impingement, corneal bearing areas, quality of peripheral and apical clearance and, generally, lens position (see Figure 4–5).

With diffuse illumination, low or high magnification, the fit of a firm corneal lens can be examined for the following:

1. *Quality of peripheral clearance.* Peripheral corneal clearance should be continuous, especially in the superior quadrants. Any discontinuity of peripheral clearance indicates corneal bearing; corneal interference is induced when a corneal lens impinges on the superior limbal areas or encroaches on the superior sclera.

Figure 4–5. Diffuse illumination, high magnification. A firm corneal lens fit for aphakia has ruptured a scleral vessel. Blood has formed on the anterior lens surface. Pigment has migrated from the iris to the posterior corneal surface and is seen at 5 o'clock. An iris vessel, the result of surgery, is seen at 3 o'clock.

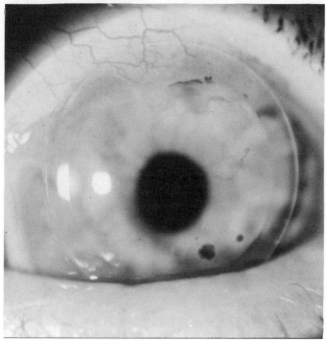

Air bubbles may be forced beneath a lens by the blink when the peripheral curves are too flat. The bubbles can stagnate and induce corneal interference. Similarly, when the peripheral curves are too steep, interference with lacrimal interchange is induced and metabolic waste may not be dissipated properly beneath the lens; gaseous bubbles form in the apical areas and create corneal interference.

2. *Quality of apical clearance.* The magnification and illumination of a biomicroscope mean less diagnostic error in the determination of apical clearance than does conventional black light fluorescein examination. The central dye patterns can be observed in greater detail with this method than with the fluorescein examination. With diffuse illumination, low or high magnification, the apical clearance areas will have various hues, according to the degree of clearance, and the apical bearing areas will be dark. Since an alignment fit is basically a *minimal apical clearance fit,* an expert diagnosis may depend on biomicroscope examination.

3. *Quantity of intermediate bearing areas.* The intermediate bearing areas will be dark. The width of intermediate zone bearing, observed with diffuse illumination, may be related to the overall lens size and the known value of the optic zone diameter. For example, if the optic zone diameter is 7.8 mm and the overall lens size is 8.8 mm, the width of the intermediate bearing area can be judged to be 0.4 mm, assuming a 0.1 mm peripheral clearance. Thus one can learn to judge how much to reduce or increase optic zone or overall lens size dimensions with this procedure.

4. *Surface wetting characteristics of a film, hydrogel, or silicone elastomer contact lens.* Surface deposits will appear either as a film that is spread across the anterior lens surface or as a coalesced group of foreign materials. One or more water droplets will gather on a corneal lens surface when the surface does not wet well. They will also form small lakes that will spread on blinking and will remain on the lens surface after blinking (see Figure 4–6).

With diffuse illumination, low magnification, the fit of a hydrogel or silicone elastomer contact lens can be examined for the following:

1. *Lens position.* Ideally, hydrogel and silicone elastomer contact lenses will have a centered position over the cornea. However, they will usually be decentered, preferably above center and in the vertical plane. They may also be decentered either tem-

Figure 4–6. Diffuse illumination, low magnification. Poor surface wetting of a gas permeable corneal lens. Water droplets form on the surface and coalesce in some areas to form lakes. Blinking will not remove them.

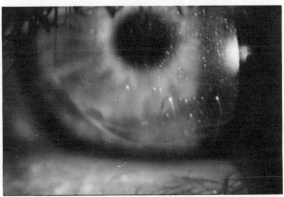

porally or nasally, but the amount of decentration must not be excessive, especially if the lens has an aspheric ocular surface, as does the Bausch & Lomb hydrogel lens. .

Aspheric contact lens surfaces become progressively flatter from the center toward the periphery and consequently show increased plus power and toroidal values from the center to the periphery. Therefore, if a lens is decentered, it will decrease the minus power needed for the distance power and will induce an astigmatic error; these factors will reduce visual acuity qualitatively and quantitatively.

2. *Lens movement.* The blink should move the lens slightly, but not excessively, to help flush corneal metabolic wastes from under the lens and create a better wearing situation. A low lens position requires a strong blinking reflex, which may be unattainable. If there is no perceptible lens movement on blinking, the fit of the hydrogel or silicone elastomer contact lens may be too secure or tight. If excessive movement occurs on blinking, the lens may be too loose.

3. *Quality of peripheral clearance.* It is difficult to assess the quality of peripheral clearance when fitting hydrogel lenses, although there may be slight blanching of conjunctival vessels when the lens is too steep. Peripheral clearance is a prerequisite for a good fit for silicone elastomer lenses.

Diffuse illumination can be used with white light, a blue filter, and fluorescein to observe the lens-cornea fit for firm corneal lenses and silicone elastomer contact lenses. It can also be used with a red-free filter for firm corneal lenses, hydrogel lenses, and silicone elastomer lenses. The red-free filter enhances the view of conjunctival and scleral vessels and of any neovascular changes induced by contact lens wear.

Direct Illumination
The most useful and most frequently employed type of illumination is direct illumination (see Figure 4–7). It is valuable for studying the cornea in detail, the characteristics of the contact lens fit, and corneal effects induced by contact lens design. Doggart wrote:

The light is directed obliquely into the eye in a beam, which, intensified by all the advantages of a dark background, illuminates brilliantly the opaque structures, and throws into relief minute optical differences in the transparent media. . . . Minute differences in the media are thus made apparent, areas of different refractivity are differentiated, and opacities of a

Figure 4–7. Direct illumination. Courtesy of Charles Erickson.

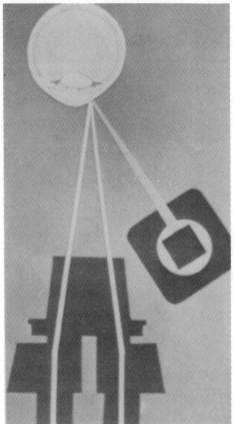

degree so slight as not to be otherwise detectable are rendered visible.[3]

Direct illumination is divided into three classifications: broad or medium beam, narrow beam, and conical beam. Each classification is designed for a different purpose (see Figure 4–8).

Regardless of the beam used, the light and the microscope are focused at the same point, the optical beam traverses the cornea obliquely, and the following things are observed:

1. The external and internal surfaces appear to be curved, since the corneal anatomy and the angle of incident light affect the degree of curvature of the arc.
2. Because there is a loss of light intensity caused by reflection, dispersion, and refraction, it is often necessary to increase illumination.

Figure 4–8. Direct illumination. (a) Diffuse illumination exposes the entire cornea. (b) The peripheral corneal areas become dark when the slit diaphragm is reduced and the illumination is changed to direct illumination, broad beam. (c) Further reduction of the slit diaphragm removes more light from the peripheral corneal areas, and the anterior and posterior corneal surfaces are exposed when the illumination is changed to direct illumination, medium beam. (ABCD represents the anterior corneal surface; EFGH represents the posterior corneal surface.) (d) An optical section is formed by direct illumination, narrow beam. (The width of the beam is 1 mm or less.) The epithelium and endothelium are not exposed in an optical section when the cornea is normal.

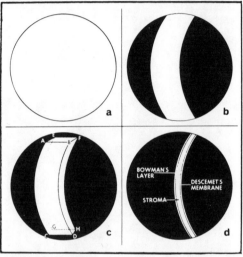

3. An optical section is formed when the width of the slit is reduced; the rectangular block formed is a parallelepiped prism.
4. The optical density of the medium is caused by the degree of relucency.

Direct illumination with broad beam and medium beam allows one to observe the quality and characteristics of the front surface of the contact lens when it is worn and to observe the fit in the apical and peripheral areas. The lacrimal flow characteristics can be observed when the incident light is changed to greater than 55°. Bubble formations beneath the lens and superficial epithelial disturbances (for example, punctates, stippling, epithelial indentation, corneal scratches, and various forms of corneal abrasions) can also be observed.

The quality of clearance areas can be assessed with direct illumination, medium or narrow beam, low and high magnification; when the tear layer is stained with fluorescein, white light or a cobalt blue filter can be used. It may be easier to judge the apparent depth of the clearance areas and the quality of the bearing areas when fluorescein is used to stain the tears, although this is not a prerequisite. The strong illumination of the biomicroscope rather than the amount of dye used probably stimulates tearing and may temporarily change the quality of the dye pool, giving rise to misleading information about the apparent depth of clearance areas.

When the light and the microscope are focused on the front surface of the dye stained tear layer, the examiner will see (1) light reflected from the front surface of the contact lens, (2) a dark area that represents the contact lens thickness, and (3) the front surface of the dye stained tear layer. The examiner should traverse the plane of the dye stained tear layer from one edge of the lens to the other to judge the apparent depth or quality of clearance or bearing in any corneal area. Clearance is represented by the full quality of the lacrimal fluid; a reduction of fluid in any area represents less clearance; corneal bearing appears as a dark, circumscribed area of no fluid. After the corneal lens is removed, the cornea can be examined in detail with this type of illumination.

Procedure for Direct Illumination, Broad Beam

For direct illumination, broad beam, make the width of the beam 2 mm or slightly more, and focus the light and the microscope on

Figure 4–9. Direct illumination, broad beam, high magnification, showing pterygium.

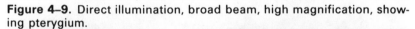
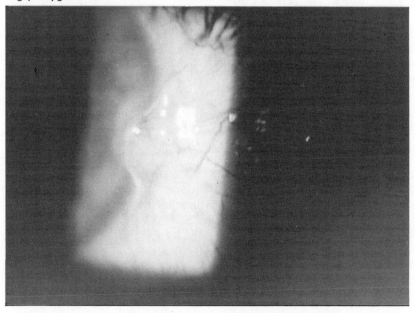

Figure 4–10. Direct illumination, medium beam, high magnification, showing penetrating keratoplasty. A conjunctival vessel encroaches on the peripheral corneal area at 3 o'clock, and a scleral vessel seems to disappear under the limbus and toward the cornea at 5 o'clock.

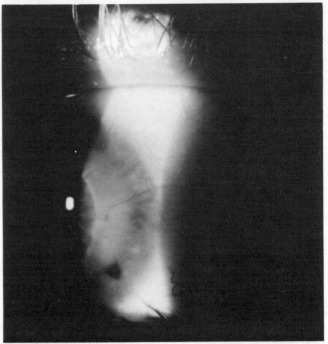

the same corneal area. Traverse the cornea from the temporal to the nasal limbal areas to examine the cornea and the contact lens fit. The anterior corneal surface and the anterior surface of the contact lens can be examined. To evaluate the contact lens fit, assess the clearance and bearing areas as well as the lacrimal flow beneath the lens. An optical section is not formed, and observation is restricted to the areas described here (see Figures 4–9, 4–10, and 4–11).

Procedure for Direct Illumination, Narrow Beam
In direct illumination, narrow beam, a further reduction in the width of the beam of direct illumination forms an optical section whereby a thin slice of tissue can be thrown into bright contrast with its unilluminated surroundings. The optical section formed is a sagittal or coronal view, not a frontal view. The optical section has been compared to a knife that cuts the tissue through its entire thickness and exposes its internal features. A thin optical section

Figure 4–11. Direct illumination, medium beam, high magnification, with the incident light beam's width between the width of the broad beam and the narrow beam. The anterior corneal surface is exposed, but the posterior corneal surface and the corneal layers are not exposed.

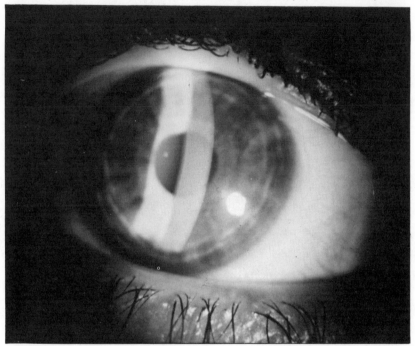

is important because it affords accurate information for diagnosis and for localization of corneal interference. The optical section (also known as the *parallelepiped of Vogt*) is always bent in the direction of the incident light, and its form varies with the angles of incidence and observation. When the slit is narrowed and the angle of incident light is 25° or greater, less of the anterior corneal surface is illuminated and corneal layers appear in section and depth. The optical section becomes a conjunctival prism when it is used to examine the limbal vessels, sclera, and conjunctiva (see Figures 4–12, 4–13, 4–14, and 4–15).

An optical section is useful and valuable for localization of depth. The stereoscopic image furnished by the microscope allows the relative position of corneal disturbance to be estimated. Superficial epithelial interferences such as punctates, epithelial indentation, stippling, and foreign bodies have a bright stain or, when fluorescein has not been used, appear without shadows on the anterior band of the parallelepiped. Objects located in the deeper corneal

Figure 4–12. Schematic drawing of the paralellepiped of Vogt and profile of an optical section.

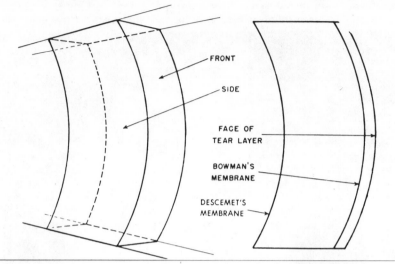

FRONT

SIDE

FACE OF
TEAR LAYER

BOWMAN'S
MEMBRANE

DESCEMET'S
MEMBRANE

layers project shadows, allowing the positions of the objects to be judged. Posterior corneal disturbances are seen on the posterior band.

The lamp and the microscope can be moved slowly over the

Figure 4–13. Direct illumination, narrow beam, low magnification. The incident light is from the examiner's right.

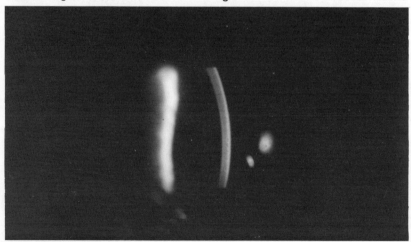

Figure 4–14. Optical section of a contact lens on the eye. (This is a biophotograph of a demonstration eye used for teaching.) Courtesy of Bausch & Lomb Corporation.

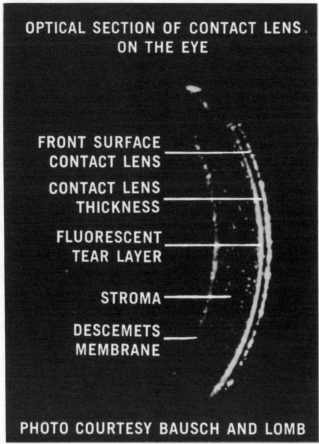

OPTICAL SECTION OF CONTACT LENS.
ON THE EYE

FRONT SURFACE
CONTACT LENS

CONTACT LENS
THICKNESS

FLUORESCENT
TEAR LAYER

STROMA

DESCEMETS
MEMBRANE

PHOTO COURTESY BAUSCH AND LOMB

cornea until the interference or object appears in the optical secton. While this is done, the variations in corneal thickness can be observed.

The technique for identifying the optical section (corneal prism) is as follows:

1. For firm corneal lenses and silicone elastomer lenses, instill one or two drops of sodium fluorescein into the eye to tint the tears green for easy identification of the anterior corneal surface. Observation can be made with or without the cobalt blue filter in place.
2. Position the lamp angle between 25° and 35° and open the slit diaphragm to establish diffuse illumination.

Figure 4–15. Optical section of a corneal lens on the eye, direct illumination, narrow beam, high magnification. The incident light is from the examiner's left. The first reflection is from the anterior surface of the contact lens. The next dark area is the lens thickness. The corneal profile is identified by the stroma that is bound anteriorly by Bowman's layer and posteriorly by Descemet's membrane. The epithelium and the endothelium of a normal cornea are not exposed by this type of illumination.

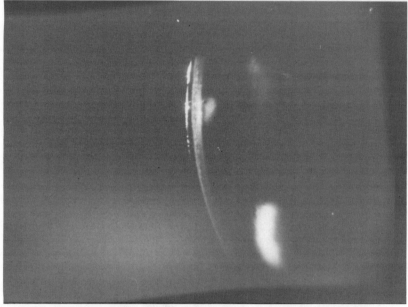

3. Slowly reduce the width of the beam to form the optical section.

Direct illumination with broad and narrow beams permits observation of the cornea, lids, conjunctiva, and sclera. It reveals contact lens surface characteristics, bubbles beneath the contact lens, and clearance and bearing areas of the contact lens on the corneal apical and para-apical zones. Direct illumination with the narrow-beam permits determination of the depth of corneal lesions.

Procedure For Direct Illumination, Conical Beam
In direct illumination, conical beam, a small circular aperture is substituted for the ordinary elongated slit when the vertical height of the slit is reduced and a concentrated pencil of light, similar to that of a searchlight, is formed (see Figure 4–16). The angle of incident light is approximately 25° to the patient's eye. The light and the microscope are focused on the patient's cornea. The vertical height of the slit is reduced by a lever on the slit lamp. When the conical beam is formed, the microscope is moved closer to the

Figure 4–16. Direct illumination, conical beam, high magnification.

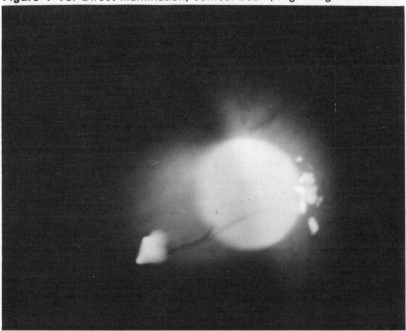

patient's eye and the beam is focused in the aqueous. Aqueous particles, if present, can be detected as they float through the conical beam; they resemble snowflakes after dark as revealed by a street lamp. Direct illumination with the conical beam permits observation of advanced turbidity of the aqueous and abnormal opalescence of the anterior chamber.

The slight flare revealed by the conical beam is physiological, although stray granules of iris pigment often float in the healthy aqueous. The conical beam has significance for discovering aqueous disturbances but has little direct relevance to contact lens practice.

According to Doggart,[4] the following abnormalities of the anterior chamber can be observed with this technique: (1) increased turbidity (flare); (2) abnormal particles—round cells (leukocytes or erythrocytes) and crystalline forms (crystals from the lens capsule); (3) heavy fluid accumulations—hyphaema (collection of blood in the anterior chamber), hypopyon (collection of pus in the anterior chamber, consisting mainly of leukocytes entangled in fibrin); (4) larger fragments—flocculent shreds (occurring in acute gonococcal iridocyclytis), detached intraocular structures (iris pigment that migrates to the aqueous after trauma), and foreign bodies (such as worms); (5) vitreous network (tremulous substance entangled in fine meshwork from subluxation of the lens and after capsulotomy); and (6) adventitious reticulation (possible sequel of interstitial keratitis, ruptures of Descemet's membrane, and fibrin accumulation on non-specific keratoiritis).

Transillumination or Retro-illumination

Illumination that requires the surface of one of the deeper structures to reflect light back toward the cornea is transillumination or retro-illumination. Light can be reflected from the iris or from the front surface of the crystalline lens; observation is slightly to the side of the reflected light. Part of the light beam that enters the eye undergoes a change in direction. One portion is absorbed by pigmented screens inside the globe, another is reflected (producing the red reflex seen in ophthalmoscopy), and the remainder re-traverses the ocular media (see Figure 4–17).

Figure 4–17. Retro-illumination and indirect illumination. Courtesy of Charles Erickson.

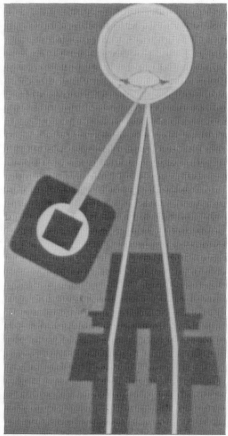

There is usually an overlap between indirect illumination and retro-illumination. For both types, the incident light is directed to the iris at an oblique angle, and, because the opaque quality of the iris allows it to serve as a reflecting screen, the cornea is illuminated from behind by the reflected light. Indirect illumination (to be discussed later) requires the light to be focused immediately adjacent to the area to be studied. When the microscope is focused on the iris, the iris is observed in direct illumination; any iritic pathological condition that lies adjacent to the directly illuminated iris portion is therefore observed with indirect illumination. The iris cannot be observed with retro-illumination (see Figures 4–18 and 4–19).

When retro-illumination is used, part of the cornea is observed by the retro method and part by the indirect. Conversely, indirect illumination of the cornea is achieved by some of the light reflected from the iris, the lens, or both. Because of this overlap, the practitioner cannot always clinically distinguish which method is actually being used at any given point in the examination.

When a corneal portion is to one side of the beam and some

Figure 4–18. Retro-illumination with light reflected from the iris exposing posterior corneal surface pigment that has migrated from the iris during cataract surgery.

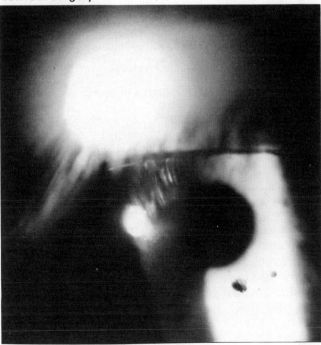

Figure 4–19. Retro-illumination, high magnification, with light reflected from the iris exposing two aperture fenestrations fabricated for a polymethylmethacrylate (PMMA) corneal lens and small bubble accumulations near the inferior limbus. Other bubbles appear in direct illumination, and a series of bubbles appear in indirect illumination in the triangular dark area between the areas exposed by retro-illumination and direct illumination. The latter may be difficult to see because indirect illumination is always proximal to the area illuminated by retro-illumination and the quality of illumination is generally poor.

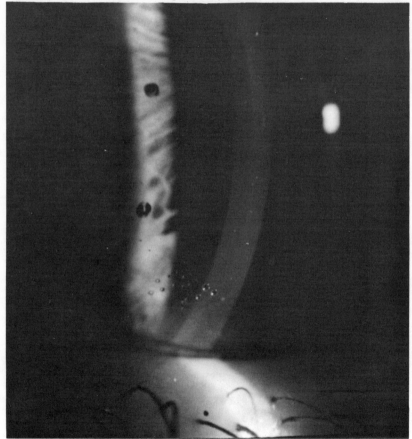

of the light reflected from the iris, the lens, or both illuminates the area of observation, color effects are created. With retro-illumination, edematous corneal epithelium will have a brownish color when the iris is brown and will appear grey when the iris is of another color. Corneal interference can be observed in the path of reflected light from the iris.

For the procedure of retro-illumination, the beam is between 1 mm and 2 mm wide and is directed to the iris or crystalline lens. The microscope is focused on the cornea, and observation is to one side of the beam of incident light. The angle of incident light and the focus of the microscope are changed to study corneal interference. When such interference is absent, there is no alteration of the normal anatomical corneal structure.

Retro-illumination permits observation of (1) corneal edema (usually of the epithelium but sometimes of all corneal layers), (2) corneal vascularization, (3) corneal lesions and deposits, (4) deposits on Descemet's membrane, and (5) abnormalities of the anterior portion of the crystalline lens.

A corneal disturbance unique to contact lens practice is a gray-white circumscribed area in the apical zone that usually corresponds to the lens position. This area can be observed, silhouetted against the dark pupil background, with various forms of biomicroscope illumination, such as sclerotic scatter and retro-illumination. Central corneal clouding is more difficult to observe when there is a small pupil diameter because it precludes sufficient background contrast. The contrast between a dark pupil background and the central corneal clouding is enhanced when the pupil is dilated.[5] Although the overall size of the affected corneal area may be related to the overall contact lens size and its optic (central) zone diameter, the size of the affected area in itself is not an indication of the severity of the condition or of the probability of a subsequent abrasion.

Central circular corneal clouding can be observed with the lens in situ; however, it is preferable to investigate its severity with the lens removed. Thus, although the diagnostic biomicroscope techniques listed here can be used for a general evaluation of the severity of the disturbance, oblique retro-illumination can be used to examine the cornea apical area in greater detail.

The practitioner should instruct the patient to gaze toward the biomicroscope's fixation light, which is placed at eye level. The slit lamp and the microscope should be coordinated in the same plane at 55° to 65° temporally. The slit lamp should be moved slowly around an arc that is never more than 10° either closer to or farther away from the patient. The position is correct when light reflected from the nasal portions of the iris illuminates the corneal apical area. It may be necessary to move the microscope stage with the joy stick to focus it on the corneal apical area. Because this procedure also moves the slit lamp and changes the angle of incident light, it is necessary to adjust the angle of incident light to correct for this factor.

The practitioner should also observe the corneal apical area in oblique retro-illumination, high magnification, for an assessment of severity. A mild edematous state appears as a series of wavy lines without form (bedewing). More advanced edema encompasses clusters of microcystic formation or irregularly shaped masses without form that may be scattered throughout the anterior corneal area. Oblique retro-illumination is used to examine the cornea for Fleischer's ring, the Hudson-Stahli line, corneal striate lines, and corneal cystic formations.

Indirect Illumination

Berliner[6] described indirect illumination as combining some features of sclerotic scatter with some of retro-illumination. Focusing a small beam on translucent tissues (for example, sclera and iris) adjacent to the area under observation allows one to see corneal features that cannot be observed with direct illumination as well as edematous areas, deep scleral vessels, iris vessels, and hemorrhages in the iris. Thus indirect illumination permits observation of part of the cornea while the light is focused on an adjacent part. Corneal interference is observed when it is adjacent to the path of reflected light from the iris.

Figure 4–20. Indirect illumination of the conjunctival and scleral vessels. An incident light beam is directed to the scleral area. The conjunctival and scleral vessels are observed in light adjacent to the incident light beam.

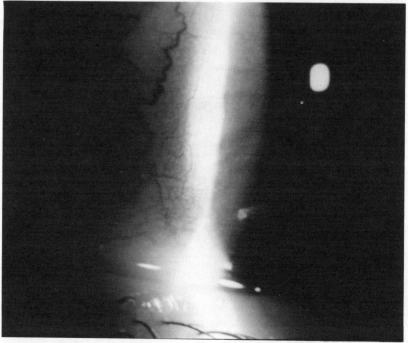

The incident light beam should be at a wide angle to the axis of observation, so that when the microscope is focused back and forth the plane of the feature under observation will be easily judged. (Oscillation of the beam permits variable illumination, which accentuates certain features perhaps overlooked in fixed illumination.) When using indirect illumination, one inadvertently swings into retro-illumination.

The procedure for indirect illumination is as follows. The beam is opened to a width of approximately 1 mm to 2 mm. The angle of incident light is approximately 60° to 70°. The light is directed to the pupil and iris. The microscope is focused on the corneal area to be studied. For observation and study of corneal interference, the angle of incident light and the focus of the microscope are changed. The area observed is adjacent to the light beam and the illuminated area. When a corneal opacity is present, there are changes in relief and three-dimensional quality (see Figures 4–20 and 4–21).

Indirect illumination permits observation of corneal lesions, opacities, deposits, surface irregularities, and vascularized areas;

Figure 4–21. Bubble formations seen in indirect illumination, high magnification, for a corneal lens too loosely fitted centrally.

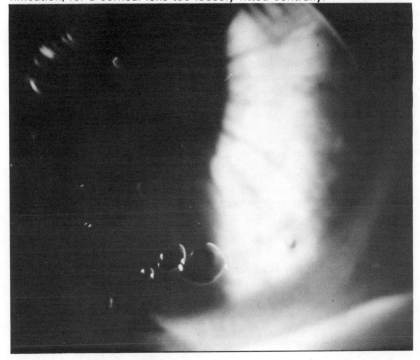

changes in the integrity of the cornea; areas of corneal edema; corneal nerves (which appear as thin white lines); wetting characteristics of the contact lens; lacrimal flow beneath the lens and movement of lacrimal debris and particles; and bubble retention and dissipation beneath the contact lens. It also permits observation of the anterior surface of the crystalline lens. (The observed orange peel effect is called shagreen.)

When indirect illumination is used and the incident light is directed to the cornea at oblique angles (between 45° and 75°), certain normal conditions as well as those indicating change may be observed. Incident light scattered obliquely through the corneal layers and across the corneal surface is a combination of scatter and indirect illumination. This approach, often called proximal illumination and sometimes referred to as an oblique form of indirect illumination, is meaningful in contact lens practice when it is used in inspecting the limbal areas for old and new vessel formation, the extreme peripheral corneal areas adjacent to the limbus for physiological edema, the superficial and deeper epithelial layers for edema, and the entire field for corneal opacities. Because incident light is reflected from the cornea at various angles, superficial corneal disturbances can be exposed by direct illumination and specular reflection.

The procedure for proximal illumination is as follows. Incident light is directed to the cornea at an angle of 45° to 75°, and the microscope is focused on the corneal surface. The angle of incident light is slowly changed by moving the light source toward 65° to 75°, and the incident light is directed to the corneal surface. The position of the microscope is changed as required to focus on the corneal or limbal areas.

Specular Reflection
Doggart,[7] Berliner,[8] and Duke-Elder[9] have described how a beam of light, when passing from one medium to another, undergoes both transmission and reflection. The amount reflected depends on the difference in refractivity between the two media. The reflection occurs at tissue surfaces, which act as mirrors, so that images of a light source are formed (regular reflection); light is also reflected from irregular polished surfaces (irregular reflection). The irregular surfaces of the epithelium and endothelium can be considered an irregular collection of minute concave and convex mirrors whose multiple images are intermingled with the larger single image of the light source seen by an observer looking in the direction of the regular reflected rays but from the opposite side, along a line

that forms an angle similar to the normal one.[10] The intensity of illumination is great and may cause patient discomfort.

Goodlaw[11] commented that specular reflection occurs when the angle of incidence equals the angle of reflection and when the microscope is directed into the reflection. The procedure is as follows. The beam is opened to a width of 1 mm to 2 mm. The angle of the lamp is set at 45° temporally, and it is moved slowly to the 90° meridian while the microscope is normal to the patient's eye and is focused on the cornea. A catoptric image of the filament is formed on the cornea; it is to the right of the incident light beam when the light is incident from the temporal section of the right eye or the nasal section of the left eye. The catoptric image is to the left of the incident light beam when the light is incident from the temporal section of the left eye or the nasal section of the right eye. The microscope is slowly moved closer to the patient's eye so that the filament of the light is in focus. At this phase of the procedure, the parallelepiped is out of focus. The beam is narrowed, and the parallelepiped is slowly moved toward the filament. The microscope is focused, and the angle of incident light is changed to expose the posterior corneal surface. (The first mirror reflection observed is from the front surface of the cornea.) When the microscope is slowly moved laterally and focused on the posterior corneal surface, suddenly the classic mosaic pattern of the corneal endothelium is exposed. The endothelium, which appears as a fine (weblike) mesh having a yellow-gold glow, is adjacent to the catoptric image of the lamp. The reflected light is very strong, and higher magnification should be used for observation and study.

Observation is restricted to a small section of the endothelial mosaic. The instrument's stage is slowly moved from side to side with the joy stick while the angle of the slit lamp is changed so as to keep the endothelial mosaic in view. The mosaic will suddenly disappear when the angles of incident and reflected light are no longer identical. It can be exposed again with the same technique when the angle of the patient's gaze is changed to a new nasal or temporal position. Observation of the endothelial mosaic is restricted to one plane; changing the height of the slit lamp changes the level of the endothelial examination.

The corneal epithelial surface and the front surface of contact lenses are examined in the zone of specular reflection. The areas of the corneal endothelium observed when the incident light is temporally directed are different from those seen with nasally directed light.

Examination in the zone of specular reflection may expose small posterior surface precipitates, which appear as black dots that mar the endothelial mosaic, looking like the defects in the silvered surface of a mirror. This type of illumination is very delicate. It is used to observe mucus and cell debris in the tears, to detect and assess changes on the anterior and posterior corneal surfaces, and to study the endothelial cells, the anterior and posterior surfaces of the crystalline lens, the shagreen effect, and the epithelial cells of the capsule. The front surface of the contact lens can be observed while the lens is being worn for irregularities such as hairline scratches, surface deposits, and poor wetting.

Oscillation

Koby[12] stated that one can have the advantage of using several types of illumination successively by displacing the illuminating lens laterally, thereby combining direct illumination, retro-illumination, and indirect illumination. The examiner oscillates the light source over an area by moving the beam of light slightly to either side. Minor changes may then become noticeable under the contrasting conditions created by rapid alternation between direct and indirect illumination. Although this technique is a practical blend of all of the methods of illumination described, it is the least used.

The procedure is as follows. For any type of illumination established, the lamp is rotated closer to and farther from the patient. Using an instrument equipped with a handle that will rotate the light beam 360°, the examiner focuses the lamp and the microscope on the cornea and moves the handle to rotate the light beam. As the light is rotated, the entire field is observed. This method facilitates further examination of the cornea and thus provides flexibility in technique. Oscillation permits observation of superficial irregularities in the corneal epithelium, corneal opacities, edematous areas of the epithelium, and small objects or filaments in the aqueous and retrolental space that might remain undetected with other forms of illumination.

Notes

1. F. E. Koby, *Slit-Lamp Examination Microscopy of the Living Eye,* trans. C. Goulden and C. L. Harris (Philadelphia: P. Blakiston's Sons, 1930).

2. J. H Doggart, *Ocular Signs in Slit-Lamp Microscopy* (St. Louis: C. V. Mosby, 1949).

3. Ibid.

4. Ibid.

5. W. G. Sampson, "Cornea Edema," in *Corneal and Scleral Contact Lenses,* ed. L. J. Girard (St. Louis: C. V. Mosby, 1967).

6. M. L. Berliner, *Biomicroscopy of the Eye* (London: Hamish Hamilton Medical Books, 1949).

7. Doggart, *Ocular Signs in Slit-Lamp Microscopy.*

8. Berliner, *Biomicroscopy of the Eye.*

9. S. Duke-Elder, ed., *System of Ophthalmology,* vol. 8 (St. Louis: C. V. Mosby, 1965).

10. Berliner, *Biomicroscopy of the Eye.*

11. E. I. Goodlaw, "Use of Slit-Lamp Biomicroscopy in the Fitting of Contact Lenses," *Encyclopedia of Contact Lens Practice* 3 (November 1961): 5–43.

12. Koby, *Slit-Lamp Examination Microscopy of the Living Eye.*

Chapter 5

Biomicroscopy for Hydrogel Contact Lenses

The development of hydrogel contact lenses excited contact lens practitioners and ametropic people because of the initial comfort of the lenses. Their water content, flexibility, "softness" implied that they would transmit oxygen in amounts that would eliminate the physical and physiological problems caused by the firm, non-gas-permeable corneal lenses.

However, practitioners have learned that soft lenses do not always eliminate corneal epithelial disturbances and edema; nor do they correct vision to the degree or quality of firm corneal lenses. Practitioners also have learned that soft lens materials are dynamic and that there must be a good lens-cornea fit, just as there is for firm corneal lenses.

A soft lens is a semiscleral lens that extends beyond the limbus to the sclera. It is more occlusive than a corneal lens, and it is in more intimate contact with the cornea. The lens-cornea fit can alter the environment of the corneal epithelial cells through changes in the tear film and at the lens-cornea interface.[1]

The initial lens-cornea fit is based on the ability of the lens polymers to absorb and hold a specific percentage of water.[2] A hydrogel lens may dehydrate from its original, fully saturated level, and the dehydration may change the base curve radius.[3] The amount of hydration is a variable for each polymer type, lens form, length of wearing time, and environmental condition.[4]

Andrasko[5] reports that hydrogel lenses begin dehydrating as they are removed from the vial and continue until a hydration equilibrium is reached on the eye. Furthermore, the time course of dehydration is mainly a function of lens thickness. Hydrogel lenses with center thicknesses of 0.07 mm and less complete their dehydration within 5 minutes of wear; those that are much thicker (for example, aphakic powers) may continue dehydrating for 30 minutes or more after insertion.

The degree of hydration established during wear varies greatly for different patients and may depend on the volume and composition of the tears. Sheridan and Shakespeare[6] believe that this is the result of the lenses, on being worn, becoming coated with some constituent of the tears that prevents or delays further water loss. The lipid layer of the tears seems the most likely to produce such a coating.

Ford[7] found an average weight loss, caused by partial hydration, of 8.79 percent after 4 hours' wear; he comments that such a loss should lead to a steepening of both front and back surface radii and an increase in the refractive index and the lens power. The mean steepening of all lenses was 0.28 mm (approximately 0.75 diopter). This is equivalent to the steepening that occurs after about 1 minute of dehydration when a fully hydrated contact lens is taken from the vial.

Dehydration may change not only the lens-cornea fit but also the surface wetting characteristics of the lens. For example, Hill has reported that the water content of hydrogel lenses may change and that the change is related to time.[8] He found that the water content for some of the lenses selected for his study was below the new lens mean while the content for others was slightly higher than average. He speculates that when water content is low, certain of the water-attracting bonding sites have been pre-emptied by contaminants building up in the lens or have been inactivated in some other way. Hill found that water content was somewhat higher in older lenses—lenses used for a longer period of time. He attributed this to a possible local weakening of the polymer structure and to laking (the formation of small, water filled cavities).

Sometimes it is necessary to add small amounts of either plus or minus spherical power to an already acceptable hydrogel lens even if there are no visible corneal changes. This need can be attributed to material changes resulting from changes in wearing conditions; it is also related to time. Janoff[9] has reported that a hydrogel lens fit can change when the lens is worn and that the changes may be caused by a drastic change in temperature and flexure. A soft lens will contract when it is dehydrated, and its contraction will cause the radii on both of its surfaces to steepen, although not always in equal amounts. This steepening can interfere with lacrimal interchange under the lens, reduce oxygen transmissivity, and induce corneal edema. Thus, a power change found when making a subjective-manifest after-refraction may also indicate the degree of corneal edema induced by the material change.

It is therefore apparent that contact lens practitioners should not expect all hydrogel lenses to retain their dimensional stability when worn. The manufacturer's specifications on the vial are dimensions at room temperature in an unstressed condition. When the lens is removed from the vial and placed on the eye, the temperature rises to 35° C and the lens is bent or draped over the cornea, which gives it a new set of dimensions.[10] Chaston and Fatt[11] list the following reasons for hydrogel lens changes on the eye:

1. Temperature changes—the temperature on the eye being higher than that in the lens vial or the room.
2. Dehydration caused by the temperature increase.
3. Change in curvature caused by fitting the lens flatter than the corneal curvature (the lens warping or draping over the corneal surface causes curvature changes).
4. Evaporation and dehydration caused by drying when the lens is worn.

The changes in lens optics and fit are a consequence of the interaction of dimensional changes brought about by all four mechanisms.

Some manufacturing changes in hydrogel lenses have simplified their fitting and have enhanced their success. For example, center thickness values have been reduced, there are fewer base curves, and the lenses transmit more oxygen. The newer, thinner, low water content hydrogel lenses should satisfy most daily wear criteria, and some of these lenses can also be used for cosmetic extended wear.

There may not be many clinical differences between some thicker hydrogel lenses made with a high water content and the thinner ones made with a low water content when both are used for either daily or extended wear and when both satisfy the cornea's need for oxygen.[12] They may also be similar in their degree of fragility, although it is sometimes more difficult for a patient to manage a thinner hydrogel lens because it folds easily.

Fitting soft lenses properly means monitoring the fit from the initial visit through the final fitting period. The final period exists when the lenses can be worn comfortably for all waking hours, without physical or physiological interference to the cornea or the bulbar and palpebral conjunctivae. It may be erroneous to assume that a soft lens is fitted properly when the patient is comfortable and satisfied with the visual correction. The dynamic properties of the material and its support of surface deposits is a major reason for continuing the biomicroscopic evaluation of the fit.

BIOMICROSCOPY OF THE EYE PRIOR TO FITTING HYDROGEL LENSES

A biomicroscope examination of the lid, palpebral and bulbar conjunctivae, sclera, and tear layer should be carried out prior to fitting any hydrogel lens, just as it is for firm corneal lenses. However, because the hydrogel contact lens is much larger than the corneal diameter and because it rests on the scleral surface, the bulbar conjunctiva and sclera should also be examined for any formations or anomalies that would preclude a good fit.

The conjunctival and scleral vessels can be examined with direct illumination, medium beam, low and high magnification, white light, and a red-free filter and with retro-illumination, low and high magnification. The vessel characteristics in the limbal areas should be examined, and a description of their extension onto the peripheral corneal areas should be recorded. The upper lid should be raised, and the superior limbal area should be examined. The upper lid should then be everted and the tarsal conjunctiva examined if the patient has worn soft lenses previously. This procedure is recommended when the soft lens use is to be changed from daily wear to cosmetic extended wear.

Direct illumination, medium beam, low and high magnification, white light, and a red-free filter can be used to examine the scleral area for elevated or xerotic areas, pingueculae, nevi, and pterygia. The slit lamp should be moved slowly from one side to the other in conjunction with the movement of the microscope's stage with the joy stick when either the temporal or the nasal scleral areas are being examined; this movement will change the angles of incident and reflected light and create other types of illumination, specifically retro-illumination and sclerotic scatter, from the scleral surface. The examination procedure, which encompasses the change from white light to the red-free filter, will enhance the observation of vascular characteristics of any elevated scleral area.

An extension of conjunctival vessels over the limbus and onto the peripheral corneal areas is generally without a consistent form and usually is less than 1 mm. Sometimes the practitioner observes a vessel that is pronounced and full and that extends from the conjunctival surface across the nasal limbal area and vertically up the peripheral corneal areas toward the superior limbal areas. This condition, along with other, similar clinical conditions that encompass the extension of conjunctival vessels onto the peripheral corneal areas, should be described and recorded for future reference.

Examining the cornea in the peripheral areas with retro-illumination will expose physiological corneal edema and conjunctival vessels that normally extend onto the peripheral corneal areas. It will also expose any unfilled vessel sheaths (ghost vessels). Some unfilled vessels sheaths are thicker than others and are therefore more easily detected. They appear as a single cylindrical form with a whitish-gray outline, and they extend toward the central corneal area.

Procedure for Observing the Cornea

1. Position the slit lamp from 15° to 20° away from the examiner.
2. Move the microscope close to the patient so that the incident light is directed to the iris at either the temporal or nasal limbal area.
3. Reduce the width of the incident light beam and establish retro-illumination at the limbus.
4. Slowly move the microscope away from the patient's eye and toward the examiner so that the retro-illumination will expose the peripheral corneal areas at the limbus.

There should be an even distribution of tears on the ocular surface when the various components of the tear film can maintain a normal tear structure.[13] The tear film is disrupted when any of these factors—the mucus, lipid, or aqueous layer of the tear film —is impaired. Persistent disruption of the tear film when contact lenses are worn may induce discomfort and preclude clinical success.

When there is an impairment in the structure of the tear film, the continuity of the dye pattern on the corneal surface will disappear and be replaced with one or more dark areas of various sizes and shapes. However, although blinking will restore the continuity of the dye pattern, the pattern will break up quickly after the blink when the preocular tear film is unstable.[14] Contact lens practitioners have traditionally used biomicroscopy to observe the breakup time (BUT) of the tear film as a way of learning if the BUT might create problems when contact lenses are worn. The obvious implication is that a condition of quantitative reduction of the tear film is a symptom of a dry eye—and that tear production is under stress.

Large molecule fluorescein is recommended for use with hydrogel lenses because the material will not absorb the dye. However, its degree of fluorescence is less than that furnished by small molecule fluorescein. It is probably preferable to use small molecule fluorescein to dye the tears and examine the corneal surface prior to fitting hydrogel lenses as a way of checking the cornea's wetting characteristics. It is also a good idea to wait until tear exchange washes the dye away or to irrigate the eye before beginning the examination with diagnostic lenses. The procedure is to place one or two drops of small or large molecule fluorescein on the scleral surface and, using diffuse illumination, low magnification, with a blue filter in the slit lamp system and a photographic yellow filter over the microscope, to focus the microscope on the corneal surface.

When the tear structure is intact, there is no interruption in the continuity of the dye patterns over the cornea. Direct illumination, medium beam, low and high magnification, with a blue filter in the slit lamp and a yellow photographic filter over the microscope is used to examine the dark areas that develop after blinking. One can count slowly (as if counting seconds), beginning immediately after the patient blinks, to estimate how long the tear structure remains intact between blinking intervals. A rapid disruption of the dye pattern continuity is an indication of poor corneal wetting.

BIOMICROSCOPY OF A SOFT LENS FIT ON THE EYE
Unlike corneal lenses made of polymethylmethacrylate (PMMA), hydrogel contact lenses use dynamic materials. The service life of these materials is undependable, although they provide a high degree of comfort. The life of a hydrogel contact lens is determined by the characteristic of surface and material changes created when they are worn.

The anterior surface of a hydrogel lens cannot sustain its optical quality because of some factors that cause its deformation. For example, eyelid pressures during blinking can cause water loss and dehydration when the material expels a small amount of water under pressure.[15] Rewetting the material allows the lens to return to its unstressed dimensions following deformation, but the degree to which it returns will critically affect its performance as a component in the optical system. This is particularly applicable to lenses made with high water uptake amounts.

Small defects, tears, cracks, and crevices in the lens are potential breeding places for bacteria and viruses and resultant lens contamination.[16] Repeated heat disinfection will cause the buildup of proteinaceous and calcareous film on a hydrogel lens.

Massaging the lens surface with a surfactant cleaner and rinsing it with saline is a way to decrease the incidence and degree of surface deposits. Such deposits are obviously a normal part of wearing soft lenses. The most we can expect, then, is to control them as much as is possible.

The methods for examining a soft lens fit biomicroscopically are identical whether they are used for diagnostic purposes, for evaluating an established wearer, or for checking on daily or extended wear. When fitting a soft lens for the first time, the practitioner can use biomicroscopy to examine the lens fit and make needed changes. Once the practitioner is satisfied with the fit of the diagnostic hydrogel lens, the patient should be instructed to wear the lens for 15 to 30 minutes so that the lens material can make a biochemical (pH) adjustment to the new on-the-eye environment. During this time the fit may change, dictating the use of another lens to create a good lens-cornea fit. Sometimes it is necessary to reduce the plus power for a lens prescribed for aphakia when the lens has equilibrated.[17]

The base curves of hydrogel lenses currently prescribed for either daily or extended wear range from 8.3 mm to 9 mm for the overall lens sizes from 13.5 mm to 14.8 mm. However, some lenses are much flatter and larger (for example, Syntex's CSI hydrogel lenses, which have a 9.35 mm base curve and a 14.8 mm overall lens size). The American Hydron Zero–4 hydrogel lens has a standard base curve of 8.7 mm; the posterior apical radii of the Bausch & Lomb Soflens varies with lens power, the base curve being on the contraocular surface.

The early soft lens forms showed a distinctive mathematical relationship between the flatter ophthalmometer corneal measurement and the lens base curve; the lens base curve was usually made 0.5 mm flatter than the flatter corneal curve. However, although hydrogel lenses are obviously fitted flatter than the flatter corneal curve, the amount of flatness is no longer emphasized. Furthermore, although practitioners may no longer select a soft lens base curve because of its mathematical relationship to the flatter corneal curvature, the relationship is still important for clinical success.

When making a biomicroscope examination of a hydrogel lens fit on the eye, the practitioner should observe and evaluate the lens for centration, position, displacement on blinking, edge fitting characteristics, surface quality, and wetting.

LENS POSITION ON THE EYE

An ideal clinical situation for a hydrogel lens fit is geometric centration over the cornea. However, the lens may be decentered either nasally, temporally, or slightly above or below the geometric center of the cornea. Sclerotic scatter, low magnification, is used to observe the lens position on the eye (see Figure 5–1).

It is easier to establish sclerotic scatter when the mirror on top of the slit lamp can be rotated. This is a characteristic of some of the older par focal instruments but not of those made with the Haag-Streit design, for which the mirror is stationary.

The following procedure can be used to create sclerotic scatter when the mirror on top of the slit lamp cannot be rotated:

1. Open the slit lamp to 1 mm or 2 mm.
2. Direct the incident light to the temporal limbal area, and focus the microscope on the temporal scleral area. The vertical illuminated slit beam on the eye will be on the cornea and will extend above and below the temporal limbal area and on the

Figure 5–1. Sclerotic scatter, low magnification.

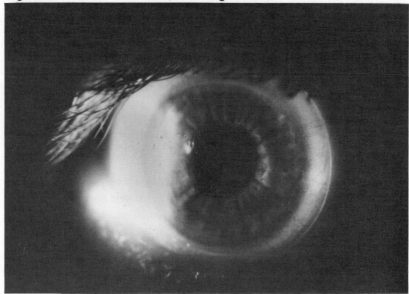

sclera in such a way that the temporal lens edge will be observed in direct illumination, medium beam; and indirect (or
trans-) illumination will illuminate the remainder of the lens
fitted on the eye.

Sclerotic scatter can be used to examine the lens position of the
eye, its displacement on blinking, and bubble formations under the
peripheral or central areas.

The slit lamp should next be positioned about 45° away from
the examiner. Diffuse illumination, low magnification, should be
used so that the incident light will make the entire lens visible.
The microscope should be focused on the lens, and the lens position
and movement on blinking should be observed. Changing to retro-
illumination will expose the bevel on the anterior surface and edge
of a Bausch & Lomb Soflens (see Figure 5–2).

A mild amount of lens displacement on blinking is preferred
because it enhances the removal of corneal metabolites and waste
products. However, normal blinking should not displace the lens
to a degree that increases lens awareness. Excessive lens movement
increases lens awareness and induces various degrees of physical
discomfort. Movement can be reduced by using a larger overall
lens size with or without a steeper base curve. However, some soft
lenses (for example, the Hydron Zero 4) are made with only one
base curve, so this technique obviously is not applicable for them.

Figure 5–2. Retro-illumination, high magnification. The bevel is on the anterior surface of a Bausch & Lomb Soflens and its edge.

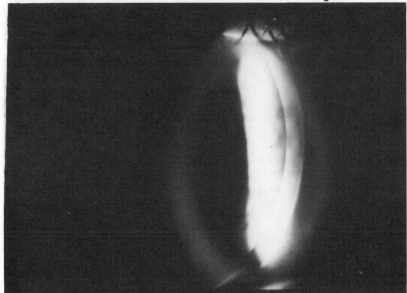

Excessive movement of a Bausch & Lomb Soflens can preclude correcting vision to acceptable levels (see Figure 5–3). The Soflens has an aspheric ocular surface that increases in plus power and radial astigmatism from the center to the periphery. An excessive amount of lens movement on blinking can cause lens awareness and visual acuity variations. Therefore, lens position and movement are meaningful criteria for this design and must be controlled to assure clinical success. The Bausch & Lomb Soflens must be made larger to reduce lens movement and improve comfort and visual acuity.

It might be helpful to place the red-free filter in the slip lamp to observe the lens position and lens displacement on blinking (see Figure 5–4). Direct illumination, medium beam, low and high magnification can be used, and the microscope can be focused on the lens edge either temporally or nasally.

The lens edge can be examined for continuity and for its relationship to the bulbar conjunctiva on blinking. For example, blinking may displace a lens with or without moving the bulbar conjunctiva. When the bulbar conjunctiva is displaced along with the contact lens, the conjunctival vessels are also displaced in the same direction. The view of the vessels can be enhanced with the red-free filter in the slit lamp.

When the overall lens is not large enough to cover the entire

Figure 5–3. Direct illumination, low magnification, showing downward displacement of a Bausch & Lomb Soflens.

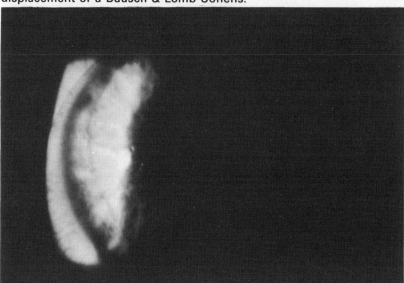

corneal diameter, the lens will move excessively on blinking. It will also overlap the limbus and rest on the sclera when the base curve is too flat and there is excessive peripheral clearance. Sometimes the upper lid will displace a loose-fitting soft lens downward on blinking. Direct illumination, medium beam, low magnification, can be used to observe the lens edge when it is displaced on blinking (see Figure 5–5).

Unlike judging a firm corneal lens fit by observing the dye patterns in the central and paracentral corneal areas, one can judge

Figure 5–4. Direct illumination, low magnification, red-free filter.

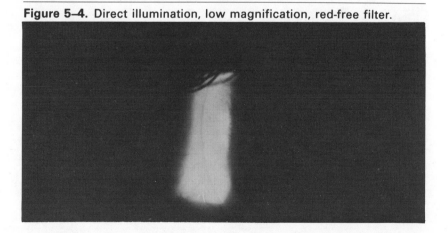

Figure 5–5. Direct illumination, broad beam, low magnification, showing excessive displacement downward on blinking for a Bausch & Lomb Soflens that is too loose.

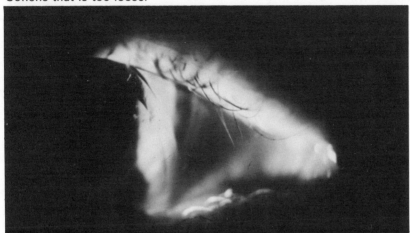

the fitting characteristics of a hydrogel lens by examining the peripheral fit. A soft lens fit is too secure when one or more bubbles (of various sizes) are trapped in the peripheral areas.

When the sagittal depth is too great, the peripheral clearance is reduced, restricting tear movement under the lens and precluding the elimination of corneal metabolic wastes. A lens with this problem should be replaced by one that has a flatter base curve. Of course, this may not be possible with a Bausch & Lomb Soflens.

The peripheral fit can be observed with direct illumination, medium beam, low and high magnification, white light, and the red-free filter. The microscope should be focused on the limbal area, and the incident light should be directed in such a way that it illuminates the limbal area and the part of the lens that rests on the sclera. A lens that fits too securely will trap one or more bubbles under it on or around the limbus and under the peripheral lens area. The location of the bubbles may be from directly under the lens edge to one or more places away from the edge and toward the limbus (see Figures 5–6, 5–7, and 5–8).

It is obvious that a new lens with a flatter base curve should be prescribed when this situation exists. Changing the base curve 0.3 mm will usually change the fit in any direction. Again, this information does not apply to the Bausch & Lomb Soflens or the Hydron Zero–4 lenses.

The lens edge will stand away from the ocular surface when the peripheral clearance is excessive. The degree and amount of edge standaway will vary, depending on the lens-cornea fit and

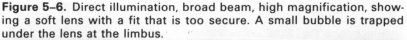

Figure 5–6. Direct illumination, broad beam, high magnification, showing a soft lens with a fit that is too secure. A small bubble is trapped under the lens at the limbus.

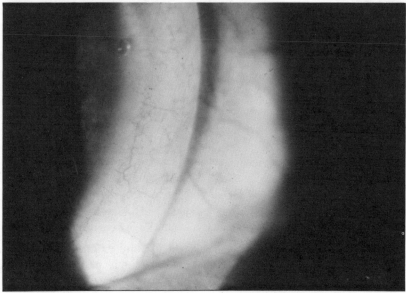

Figure 5–7. Direct illumination, broad beam, high magnification, showing a soft lens with a fit that is too flat. A large bubble under the lens is caused by lens edge standoff.

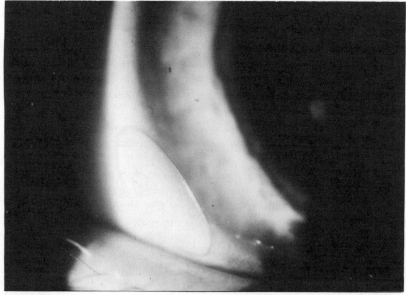

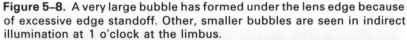

Figure 5–8. A very large bubble has formed under the lens edge because of excessive edge standoff. Other, smaller bubbles are seen in indirect illumination at 1 o'clock at the limbus.

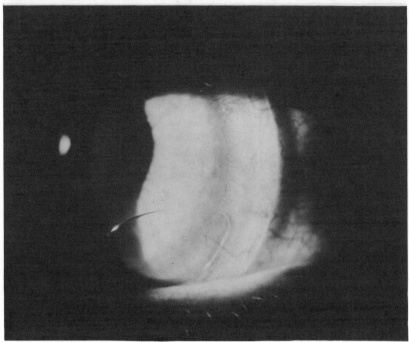

the ability of the material to retain its hydrated state. A diagnostic lens fit may seem fine on initial observation but may change when the lens has equilibrated.

The lens will stand away from the ocular surface in the periphery when the base curve is too flat, water is lost by evaporation, and the lens becomes dehydrated. (The latter situation may develop more frequently when soft lenses are used for cosmetic extended wear than when they are used for daily wear.)

Direct illumination, medium beam, low and high magnification, can be used to examine the continuity of the lens edge on the scleral surface. There will be a loss of circular continuity when the lens edge is affected by dehydration (see Figure 5–9).

The incident light can be made wider or narrower as needed to observe the characteristics of edge fit. Increasing the width of the incident light to direct illumination, wide beam, low and high magnification, will expose edge curling or liftoff from the ocular surface (see Figure 5–10).

It is rare for the patient to be aware of a change in the fit of the lens when the degree of edge lift is relatively small. However,

Figure 5–9. Examination of a soft lens edge. An interruption of circular continuity of the edge occurs at 1 o'clock.

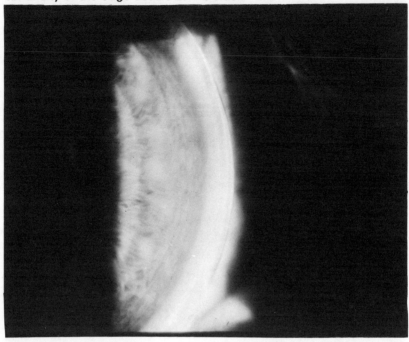

Figure 5–10. Small amount of edge curling.

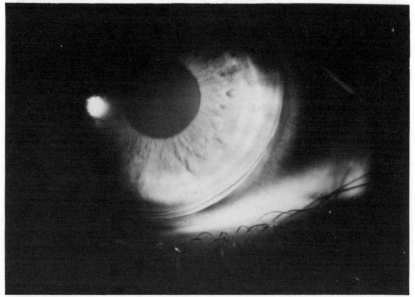

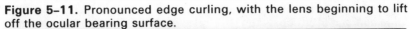

Figure 5–11. Pronounced edge curling, with the lens beginning to lift off the ocular bearing surface.

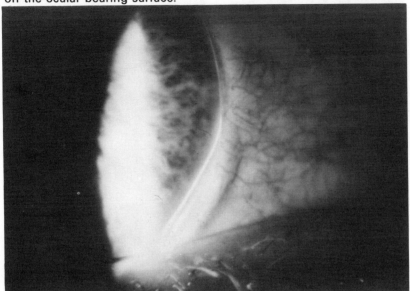

there is a progressive increase in lens awareness as the degree of edge lift increases (see Figure 5–11). When the peripheral fit is excessive, the lens edge will lift off the ocular surface and curl away from it. Retro-illumination, low or high magnification, can be used to examine the characteristics of edge lift or edge curl. In Figure 5–11, specular reflection from the affected area enhances its appearance.

When the surface of a hydrogel lens is examined with direct illumination, medium and wide beam, low and high magnification, the incident light may expose poor wetting of the lens surface in specular reflection (see Figure 5–12). Edge curl and liftoff can be observed with retro-illumination and indirect illumination that is secondary to the primary type of illumination selected.

When there is excessive peripheral clearance, the upper lid can grasp the lens, raise it, and lift it off the ocular surface and over the top of the lower lid (see Figure 5–13). This clinical situation, observed in diffuse illumination, high magnification, obviously indicates a poor fit, and the lens should be replaced with one made with a steeper base curve or having a larger overall size.

Spincasting, molding, and lathing are the methods used to manufacture hydrogel lenses. It is imperative that lenses made by lathing have smooth, unblemished surfaces. Although it is rare, lenses sometimes pass inspection with tool (lathing) marks remaining on the anterior surface.

Figure 5–12. Poor wetting of the lens surface seen in specular reflection. Edge curl and liftoff observed with retro-illumination and indirect illumination.

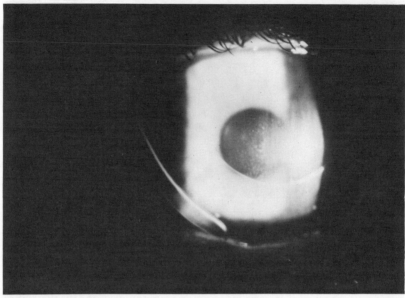

Figure 5–13. Diffuse illumination, high magnification, showing excessive peripheral clearance. The upper lid has grasped the lens, raised it, and lifted it over the top of the lower lid.

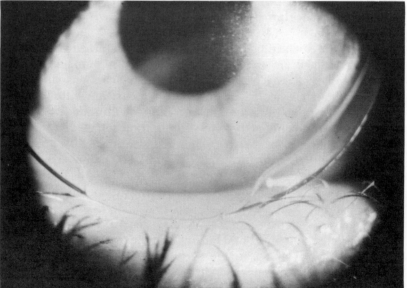

Figure 5-14. Retro-illumination, low magnification, showing structural changes—a series of irregular vertical linear formations caused by dehydration—in a hydrogel contact lens.

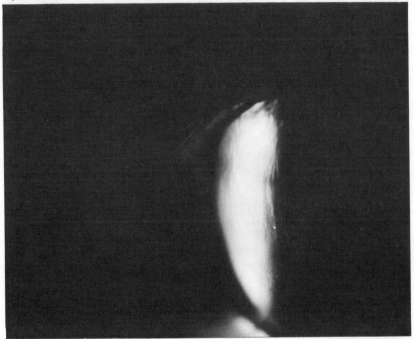

Direct illumination, medium and broad beam, low and high magnification, white light, is used to examine the lens surface for optical quality and surface defects. Tool marks appear as one or more irregular linear formations. They are usually superficial, and it is rare for their presence to create physical discomfort. However, the lens should be replaced when a biomicroscope examination exposes such marks.

Structural changes in a hydrophilic lens can be detected with direct illumination, medium beam, low and high magnification. The lens will look wrinkled, and it may or may not induce physical discomfort and visual acuity changes (see Figure 5-14). The lens should be replaced, and the cornea should be examined for such edematous changes as microcystic formations. Small or large molecule fluorescein can be used to stain the tears when the lens is removed and to examine the corneal surface for epithelial staining and wetting characteristics.

Crazing or cracking of the surface of a hydrophilic lens may occur when the lens becomes partially or completely dehydrated.[18] This surface defect can be seen with direct illumination, medium

Figure 5–15. Crazing or cracking of the surface of a hydrophilic contact lens.

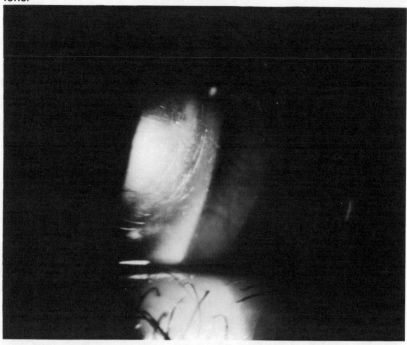

Figure 5–16. Foreign material in a hydrogel contact lens.

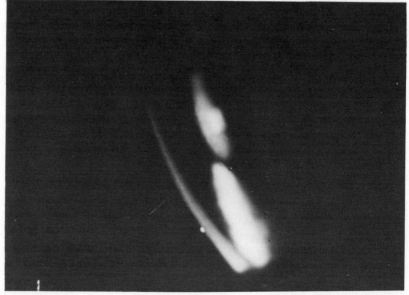

and broad beam, low and high magnification. It appears as a series of irregular circular formations (see Figure 5–15).

Occasionally, one or more red spots can be found in hydrophilic lenses. Bier and Lowther[19] state that the spots are apparently areas of rusted iron oxide or steel that are on the surface of or embedded in the lens. These circular, orange-colored particles are usually superficial and are observed with direct illumination, low and high magnification (see Figure 5–16).

The practitioner should also use the biomicroscope to examine the lens edge for nicks and tears. A lens may have a torn edge without creating physical discomfort or even awareness in the wearer. Much of this damage is caused by the cases used for hydrogel lens storage, particularly those that have a perforated lid attached to the semihemisphere used to hold the lens in the case. A torn or damaged hydrogel lens edge can be observed with direct illumination, medium beam, low and high magnification (see Figure 5–17). The incident light beam can also be displaced to the right or left of the damaged edge so the edge will be illuminated in retro-illumination. Although the damaged edge illustrated in Figure 5–17 is obvious, sometimes there is only a series of small contiguous nicks on the lens edge; such nicks have a serrated appearance. Also, there may be a rupture, or slight tear, in the main body of the lens. Regardless of the location of the physical damage to the lens, it

Figure 5–17. Torn soft lens edge.

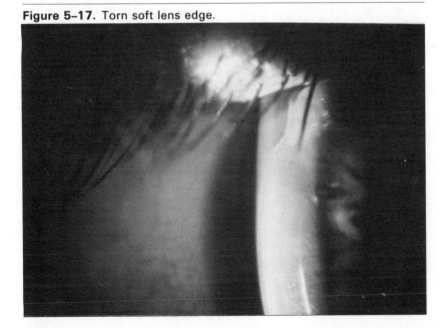

is rare for the patient to be aware of it; the practitioner must therefore bring it to the patient's attention.

SOFT LENS SPOILAGE

A good fit may become a poor one when there is either a structural change that changes the lens-cornea by interfacing with the normal corneal physiological state or lens surface spoilage. As for the clinical problems created by lens changes, the development of surface changes is the more common and may dictate a need to replace the lens.

Contact lens practitioners must depend on conventional biomicroscopy to detect and evaluate surface deposits. Unfortunately, conventional biomicroscopy restricts the observation to the lens surface. Other forms of examination, such as phase contrast microscopy, specular microscopy, and scanning electron microscopy, are more extensive and revealing; thus a more definitive diagnosis and evaluation of lens spoilage can be made with them.

Conventional biomicroscopy can be used to detect surface deposits and study them with respect to their size and color.[20] Phase contrast microscopy can be used to examine lenses for surface problems such as breaks, deposits, and manufacturing defects.[21] Practitioners who have investigated lens spoilage with these various microscopic methods in addition to conventional biomicroscopy have come to similar and, in some instances, identical conclusions about the etiology and identification of the chemistry of surface deposits. For example, some believe that crevices and cracks on the surface are lathe markings that have been insufficiently polished.[22] Others postulate that lens scratches are caused by dessication, by detached granular deposits that rub against the lens surface with the movements of the eyelids, or by daily cleaning when the lenses are rubbed with the finger.[23]

The specular microscope normally is used to examine the endothelium. However, Rao and his colleagues[24] used the newly developed Keeler specular biomicroscope to observe spoilage of soft contact lenses while the lenses were on the eyes. They were able to identify surface and edge defects, mucolipoproteins, and inorganic deposits. Rao believes that specular microscope examination of a soft contact lens on the eye will show lens spoilage at an earlier stage than is possible with the conventional biomicroscope.

Surface deposits are indigenous for hydrogel contact lens materials. Their incidence and degree are variable and unpredictable. They directly affect the comfort, visual acuity, wearing time, and service life of the lens. Various etiologies may account for differences in the shape, color, texture, and geometry of such deposits. It appears that the deposits are the result of chemical changes on the lens surface and that they cannot be controlled by changing contact lens management methods for asepticizing, storing, cleaning, and using solutions on the lenses.

Morgan[25] reports that there is no established relationship for cause, incidence, and degree between the types of surface deposits found and the contact lens materials. As for specific clinical situations that deal with surface deposits, he found that (1) the incidence of calcium deposits was greater for people in the older age groups, (2) the incidence of surface deposits for hydrogel lenses with relatively low water content was less than that for higher water content materials, and (3) protein deposits were more prevalent for the low water content materials.

Morgan[26] also found that cleaning hydrogel lenses with enzyme cleaners changed the lens fitting characteristics; 15 percent of such lenses functioned differently after enzyme cleaning. Morgan reported that enzyme cleaning created physical discomfort and loss of centration and left remnants of the deposits, such as lipids and cholesterol. The lipid and cholesterol deposits caused the lens edges to dry rapidly and lift off the ocular surface.

Morgan also investigated blood chemistry levels to learn if they could be related to lens coating. He found that blood cholesterol levels were indeed linked to lens coating as well as to changes in lens absorbance, transmittance characteristics, and relationships with lipid deposits. Morgan concluded that contact lens wearers with higher than normal levels of alkaline phosphatase and cholesterol have a greater incidence and degree of lens coating. He also noted that the deposits on hydrophilic lens surfaces are proteins and lipids and that, unexpectedly, enzyme cleaning does not remove all the surface deposits.

Bier and Lowther[27] refer to a change in surface texture as well as to the age and deterioration of the material itself as a possible etiological factor. This situation can be attributed to prescribing lenses that have been used as diagnostic lenses many times so that the patient's lenses are not really new, having been used and handled previously. All the descriptions of poor clinical situations for hydrogel lenses with surface deposits assume that the lenses prescribed for patients have never been worn before. Unfortunately, this is not always true, especially when practitioners have large amounts of inventory on consignment. They may use the same materials for several patients in making clinical investigations and then may prescribe one of the "used" lenses for a patient.

Hathaway and Lowther[28] found no correlation between protein concentration and the rate at which deposits accumulated; however, they did find a correlation between the deposit rate and both the Schirmer test and breakup time. A short BUT was correlated with a rapid deposit formation.

It is obvious that surface deposits reduce wettability and may lead to lens rejection. An anachronism is described by Tighe,[29] who stated that the more wettable the surface, the more the surface will promote adhesion of materials that will eventually reduce the wettability.

The majority of soft lens deposits observed with biomicroscopy seem to be derived from ocular secretions in the tears. Tripathi and Ruben[30] describe the following derivation of soft lens deposits:

1. Proteinaceous deposits occur when the pH of the tears is low.
2. Mineral deposits occur when the pH of the tears is high.
3. Gelatinous deposits form when the lenses are not cleaned properly before heat asepticizing. They may also be caused by dry spots.
4. Birth control pills can cause abnormal mucin formations.
5. Lipid formations are due to a combination of dryness and stress on the lens from blinking. Blinking alters the structural integrity of the lens surface so that a lipid coating from the Meibomian gland secretion can form.
6. No definitive causes are known for calcium formations, although the authors suggest several possibilities.
7. Various extraneous factors exist. Among them are (a) finger dirt, cosmetics, and ocular medications; (b) mechanical stress caused by rubbing, handling, entropion, and so on; (c) environmental factors such as rust spots; (d) microbial contamination that can result from heat disinfection; and (e) manufacturing defects.

The lens deposits can induce refractive changes and changes in the corneal physiology, such as superficial punctate keratitis, dry spots, edema, and dilation of superficial pericorneal vessels. Some related changes are giant papillary conjunctivitis and neovascularization. Ocular infections and uveitis are other related but rare changes.[31]

Surface deposits were observed on hydrophilic contact lenses soon after practitioners began to fit them.[32] However, their identity was established when Karageozian successfully identified the deposits as protein and hypothesized that lysozyme was a major cause of them. Previously the deposits had been identified as lipid and calcium as well as protein. The development and use of a commercial papain-containing cleaning product for the digestive removal of these protein deposits along with improvements in surfactant cleaners have extended the service life of hydrophilic contact lenses, but no improvements have eliminated the problem of surface deposits and resultant lens spoilage.

Feldman[33] comments that hydrophilic lenses have highly reactive surfaces and that the same functional groups that are used in binding water will also become binding sites for proteins and inorganic ions. He further states that the protein deposits on a soft lens surface provide a secondary binding site for other substances. Thus there is a constant effort to control the interaction between tear proteins and the lens surface and thereby limit the degree of lens spoilage caused by surface deposits. Thermal and chemical disinfection methods, patient negligence in following instructions,[34] and agents found in contact lens solutions.[35] have been proposed as possible etiological factors for the development of surface deposits.

How meaningful are surface deposits in the successful wearing of hydrophilic contact lenses? Hill[36] reported that as the degree of spoilation advances, oxygen performance values decline. Consequently, for very thin hydrogel lenses, especially those that are prescribed for cosmetic extended wear, an advanced state of surface deposits will not allow the lens to maintain its full capacity of energy reserves.[37] Any lens change that interferes with the physical and physiological fit can change a good fit to a poor one by inducing physical discomfort and a reduction in visual acuity. Unfortunately, surface deposits may be beyond the control of contact lens practitioners, who can only depend on a biomicroscope examination of the lens fit on the eye to detect the deposits and manage the problems they cause.

Biomicroscopy can be used to examine a lens surface on the eye with direct illumination, indirect illumination, specular reflection, and retro-illumination. Visible changes include material discoloration, poor surface wetting and dry spots, surface irregularities, edge defects, and focal, discrete, or diffuse deposits (for example, proteinaceous, gelatinaceous, lipoidal, calcreous, mulberrylike configurations, concretions, and cellular, lycelial, and cystic changes).

Diffuse illumination, low magnification, should be used to observe the surface wetting characteristics of a hydrogel lens. The patient should be instructed to blink normally while observing the lens on the eye. The lens surface will become wet on blinking and may quickly begin to dry in one or more areas when the lids open between blinks. The nonwet areas have a dull appearance where the drying occurs and resemble a film that seems to spread rapidly over the area as it dries. Although this drying may imply that the patient will have problems wearing hydrogel lenses, it could also be caused by a poorly fabricated surface. Therefore, when this situation occurs with a diagnostic lens, the lens should be replaced with another one of identical values to see if the poor wetting is caused by a poor lens surface or the inability of the patient's tears to keep the lens surface wet. When drying is found in the lenses of established wearers, it may be caused by lens spoilation.

The anterior lens surface will lose its apparent transparency in a poor wetting area. Such an area on the lens surface has a bright gray-white appearance when viewed with specular reflection. It first appears as a confluency of several small circular particles from the tears that begin to evaporate quickly. Although a poor wetting area observed with specular reflection seems dense or thick, this characteristic changes when it is observed with direct illumination, medium or narrow beam; the area then may appear less dense or thick. Scattered irregular gray-white linear forms resembling corneal edema can be seen with direct illumination, medium beam, low and high magnification. Generally, surface deposits have a representative size, are without regular form, and can be found at any location on the surface.

An alternate procedure is to use direct illumination and retro-illumination, low and high magnification, to examine the character-

---

Figure 5-18. Direct illumination, medium beam, high magnification, showing a rupture in the mucin layer of the tears.

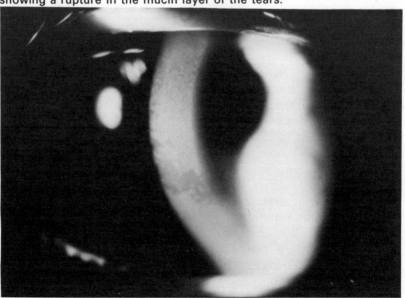

istics of surface deposits for their location, size, and depth. Also, the lens surface and the lens material should be examined for defects such as rust particles, surface linear formations, and edge lift.

Contact lens wearers depend on frequent blinking and a good tear supply to keep the lenses wet. Any defect in the tears or the lens surface can create wearing problems.[38] A quick rupture of the mucin layer of the tears is a potential problem source; it can be observed in white light using direct illumination, medium beam, low and high magnification (see Figure 5–18).

Particles or debris in the tears can be observed with diffuse illumination, low and high magnification (see Figure 5–19). Defects in the tear layer may preclude easy movement of the lids over the ocular surface, decrease the mucoprotein content of the precorneal tear film, and change the surface tension. The patient should be informed that a tear film defect could cause a fitting problem, and the practitioner should proceed with the fitting only when the patient understands this problem. Fortunately, few candidates for soft contact lenses have failed to be fitted because of defects in the tear layer.

Lens surface spoilage may begin as a series of small, circular gray-white deposits scattered on the lens surface and seen with diffuse illumination, low and high magnification. The microscope is focused on the deposits, which are so small that they will not

Figure 5–19. Debris in the tear layer.

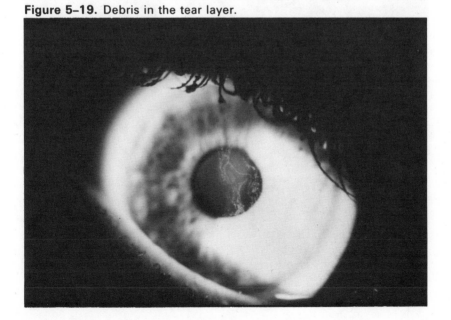

intefere with vision or comfort. The deposits can be examined further with direct illumination, medium and narrow beam, low and high magnification, and sclerotic scatter, low magnification. When the deposits are detected, the lens should be removed and cleaned with a surfactant cleaner and rinsed with a saline solution before wearing is resumed. However, surface deposits will return, and as the degree of lens surface spoilage increases, they will become larger, thicker, and more uncomfortable.

Several researchers have reported that because of the complexity of ocular physiology, the composition of deposits and coatings varies; some such deposits may have a crystalline structure resembling that of mineral deposits such as calcium.[39] Calcium deposits on a soft lens surface are seen in direct illumination, wide beam, low or high magnification. They appear as discrete circular, white, opaque surface deposits (see Figure 5–20). Hathaway and Lowther[40] comment that the calcium for these deposits appears to be derived from either the physiological precorneal tear film or the solutions for normal lens care. The increased use of distilled water and salt tablets may be responsible for some calcium deposits on the soft lens surface. Therefore, Lowther and Hathaway recommend that

Figure 5–20. Discrete opaque surface deposits on a hydrogel lens.

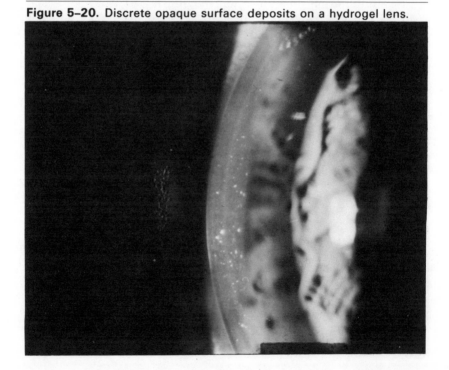

those who use salt tablets to prepare their saline solutions should use only high-quality (USP) distilled water in formulating the solutions.

It is obvious that hydrogel lens surfaces have an affinity for foreign material of various descriptions. Yet the lens surfaces wet well and are clear when they are worn for the first time. Thus the sequential clinical development of surface spoilage makes it appear that hydrophilic sites develop on the lens surface regardless of the etiological factors and that the loss of hydrophilic properties begins in one area and expands to others.

A relatively thin surface film may cover a part of the lens surface (seen in specular reflection immediately after blinking) and is obviously a poor surface wetting condition (see Figure 5–21). In fact, the film does not cover the hydrophobic area completely; there are scattered places within its borders where the deposit has not formed on the lens surface. There is also a single circular calcium deposit that has formed on the surface in the area covered by the film. The patient will report visual distress and lens discomfort when this deposit is present. The lens should be removed, cleaned, and returned to the eye. It must be replaced with another lens if cleaning does not restore visual acuity and comfort.

Surface deposits may first appear as a film or a series of discrete

Figure 5–21. Specular reflection from a hydrogel lens surface, showing a surface film on the lens and poor wetting.

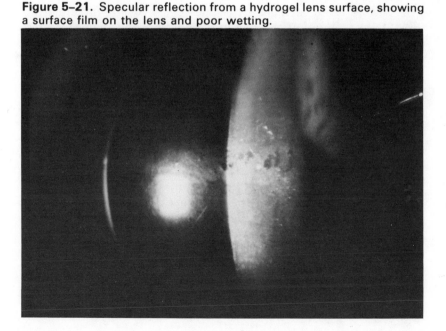

Figure 5–22. Specular reflection from a hydrogel lens surface, low magnification, showing an accumulation of small, circular, opaque white surface deposits.

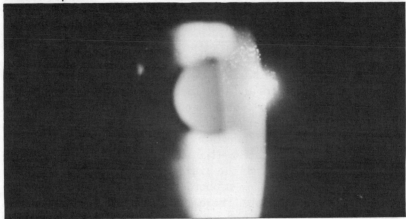

small, circular, white formations in the paracentral lens area located near the pupil; they are easily detected with specular reflection (see Figure 5–22). The lens should be removed, cleaned with a surfactant cleaner, rinsed with saline, and returned to the eye. Newly formed deposits are easily removed, but the practitioner should continue to use biomicroscopy to observe the lens surface to learn if the deposits will recur.

The scattered particles may coalesce and cover a larger surface area. Direct illumination, medium beam, low and high magnification, is used to detect and examine the deposit (see Figure 5–23). The specular reflection also present highlights much of the detail or structure of the deposit.

A larger surface area is covered when the size of the surface deposit increases. Direct illumination, broad and medium beam, low and high magnification, is used to examine the deposit and the surrounding area. Specular reflection is included in the observation as the angle of the slit lamp and incident light is changed to enhance the observation (see Figure 5–24). The width of the incident light is decreased to form direct illumination, narrow beam, low and high magnification, so that the deposit can be examined for its thickness (see Figure 5–25). An increase in the size and thickness of a surface deposit can cause the upper lid to grasp the lens and displace it (see Figure 5–26).

Using specular reflection to examine surface deposits will make it easier to recognize the quality and form of the deposits. A distinction can be made between their elevated areas and form and their typical dull, dense, irregular deposits that the elevated areas cover.

Figure 5–23. Coalesced surface deposits.

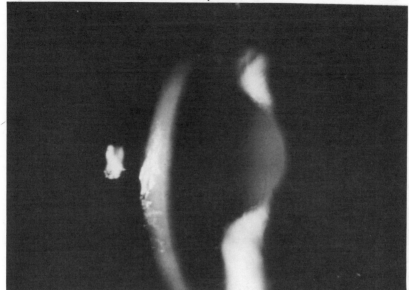

Figure 5–24. Surface deposits on a soft lens surface.

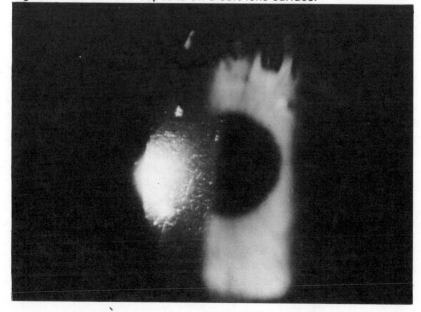

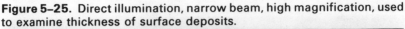

Figure 5–25. Direct illumination, narrow beam, high magnification, used to examine thickness of surface deposits.

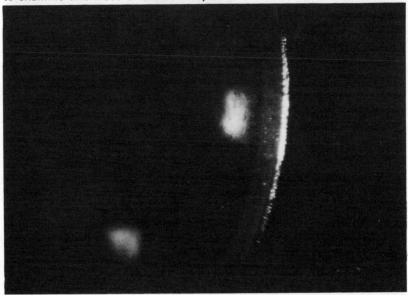

The lens with surface deposits should be removed, cleaned with a surfactant cleaner, rinsed with saline, and replaced on the eye. Surface deposits are easily removed when they are relatively simple (for example, composed of scattered particles or not very thick). A large, thick lens should be immersed in a beaker containing 3 percent hydrogen peroxide and should then be placed in an ultrasonic cleaner for 10 minutes. After the ultrasonic cleaning, the lens should be placed in another beaker containing a saline solution and then should be put in the ultrasonic cleaner for 20 minutes of further agitation and rinsing. Although this is a way to remove surface deposits, good vision and comfort will not be restored if the debris has been absorbed into the lens matrix, a clinical situation that cannot be detected with a conventional biomicroscope. Therefore, when ultrasonic cleaning has been used, the lens should be replaced on the eye and examined with a biomicroscope to confirm the removal of surface deposits; then the patient's vision should be recorded. The cleaning is effective when it restores visual acuity and comfort. The lens must be replaced with a new one if the cleaning removes the surface deposits but does not restore vision.

An interesting type of surface deposit is one that resembles a gelatinous mass. It is a circular formation, transparent or translucent, that may exist either alone or in conjunction with other types of surface deposits. When it is a single entity, it is easily removed

Figure 5-26. Thick surface deposit and displacement of a soft lens.

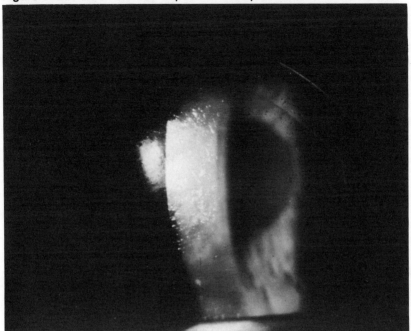

with a surfactant cleaner. A gel deposit is elevated and can fasten itself to any place on the lens surface. It is easily detected with direct illumination, medium beam, low and high magnification (see Figure 5-27) and can be studied further with retro-illumination, low and high magnification (see Figure 5-28).

In Figure 5-29, an elevated single gel deposit at the lens surface is juxtaposed with a coalesced surface deposit. The method of illumination is direct illumination, medium beam, although specular reflection from the coalexced area obscures the form and detail of the area. The gel deposit is seen in retro-illumination at 11 o'clock at the pupil margin. In Figure 5-30, a cluster of gel deposits is seen in indirect illumination, although specular reflection highlights some of it.

Lens spoilage can also encompass absorption of foreign material that decreases visual acuity and comfort. Conventional biomicroscopy does not detect this condition; practitioners must therefore rely on the patient's subjective symptoms to determine that it exists and is responsible for a clinical problem.[41] If replacement of the uncomfortable lens with one having identical parameters restores vision and comfort, then the diagnosis is confirmed.

Another form of lens spoilage is a structural change created

Figure 5–27. Gel deposit seen in direct illumination, medium beam.

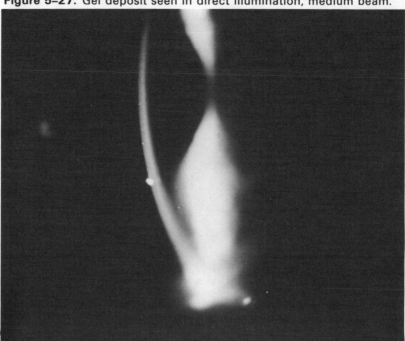

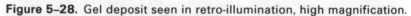

Figure 5–28. Gel deposit seen in retro-illumination, high magnification.

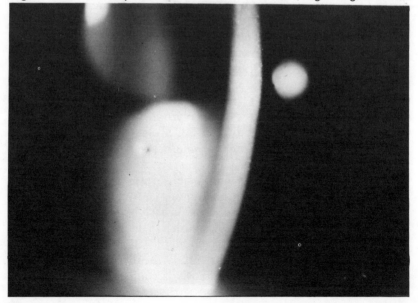

Figure 5-29. Gel deposit seen in retro-illumination and other surface deposits seen in specular reflection.

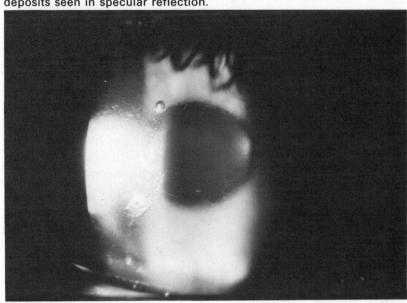

Figure 5-30. Cluster of gel deposits.

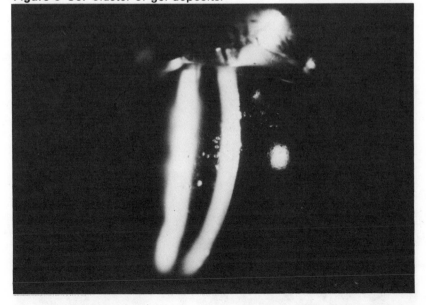

by lens evaporation and dehydration.[42] The lens fit becomes more secure when the lens dehydrates. This clinical situation is most prevalent among those who wear hydrophilic lenses for cosmetic extended wear.

When the lens dehydrates, a series of small bubbles accumulate behind it and the lens-cornea fit becomes more secure. The bubbles are easily detected with a biomicroscope; they are observed with direct illumination, medium beam, and retro-illumination, low and high magnification. They are not very large, but they seem to form clusters (see Figure 5–31). One can use small molecule fluorescein on the sclera or on the inferior palpebral conjunctiva to stain the tears and direct illumination, broad beam, with the blue filter to observe the lens fit. The hydrophilic lens have corneal clearance and corneal bearing at the limbal area. The bubble clusters at 8 o'clock are not moved on blinking. Similarly, the scattered bubbles found under the lens are stationary, implying that the lens fit has become more secure.

In Figure 5–32, the lens has been removed and the bubbles have indented the corneal epithelial area where they were retained. There is no pain or discomfort when the lens is worn or when it is removed. The bubbles may be an intracellular collection of fluid or small vacuoles that have migrated to the surface, where they are retained by the lens.[43] Replacing the lens with one having identical parameters will restore vision and comfort when the physical change in the lens-cornea fit has been caused by dehydration.

Figure 5–31. Bubble accumulations under a soft lens seen in retro-illumination at 7 o'clock at the pupil border.

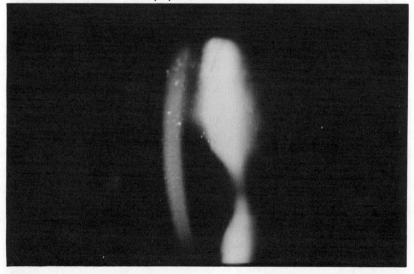

Figure 5–32. Corneal epithelial indentations, or dimpling, caused by bubble retention under a soft lens.

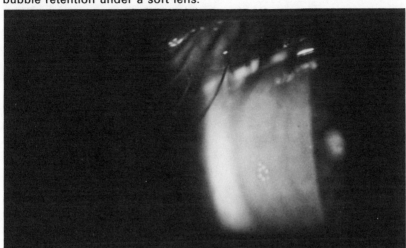

BIOMICROSCOPE EXAMINATION OF THE EYE WHEN SOFT LENSES ARE REMOVED

Hydrogel lenses are classified according to their water content, oxygen transmissivity, and prescription for daily or extended wear. In fact, some contemporary single vision hydrogel lenses can be used for both daily and cosmetic extended wear because they transmit oxygen in amounts that can satisfy both modalities.

The introduction of thin and ultrathin hydrogel contact lenses has simplified fitting and reduced the incidence and degree of fitting problems.[44] The lenses take less time to reach an equilibrium, their greater flexibility leads to a better molding effect, and a given lens will fit a wider range of corneal shapes. These lenses provide improved physical comfort; they also reduce fitting time, lid feel, lens awareness, poor centration caused by asymmetric or flat corneas, and the incidence and degree of corneal edema.

In regard to the oxygen levels required by the cornea to maintain its transparency, low water content thin hydrogel lenses are satisfactory for daily wear and for extended periods of consecutive overnight wear when the lens-cornea fit is good. Benjamin and Hill[45] have calculated that a HEMA lens of 0.06 mm center thickness would have an EOP value of 7 percent. This value is well above the edema threshold, even leaving the energy reserves intact. Hill and Mauger[46] have reported an EOP of 9.4 percent for production spuncast HEMA lenses of 0.035 mm center thickness.

Contact lens practitioners must rely on the information printed on the soft lens vials along with the description of the physiochemical properties of the lens material furnished by the manufacturer as a way to estimate the clinical performance of a hydrogel contact lens selected for either daily or extended wear. However, it does not always follow that a hydrogel lens will perform as expected; therefore, clinical problems develop.

Oxygen transmitted by a hydrogel contact lens is determined by the equation Dk/L, where Dk is oxygen permeability and L is the center thickness of the lens. Refojo[47] observed that as the water content in hydrogels increases, so does the oxygen permeability— and in a fairly predictable progression.

Flynn, Quinn, and Hill[48] explored this assumption further by dividing the water content (which tends to raise oxygen performance) by the center thickness (which tends to lower oxygen performance); they called the quotient the hydration to thickness (H/T) index. The assumption they made was that the larger the H/T index, the more oxygen should pass through the lens. Their investigation confirmed that the mathematical calculation is one thing and the clinical performance of a given material is another. Several factors combined to influence the clinical performance of a hydrogel material so that it did not always perform as expected on the basis of the H/T index. These factors are the fullness of hydration of a material as it is being worn, the effects of acidity on water content (and thus on oxygen permeability), and other polymer peculiarities.

Consequently, contact lens practitioners should have those who wear hydrogel lenses return to their offices at frequent intervals for perfunctory biomicroscope examinations of the contact lens fit on the eye and of the eye itself when the contact lens is removed. Patients who use hydrogel lenses for daily wear might return every 3 months; those who use the lenses for extended wear might return every 2 months. Although these returns will increase office traffic, they are an excellent way to confirm the efficacy of a fit and to intercept problems.

The ideal sight vehicle for an ametropic person is one that will correct vision for extended periods without removal. Such a vehicle must maintain the oxygen levels of the cornea that are required for normal corneal thickness. Fatt and Freeman[49] have calculated that the closed eye receives about 7 percent EOP. Hill[50] has suggested that an arbitrary safe minimum is 11 percent.

Although ultrathin low water content soft contact lenses can be prescribed for either daily wear or extended periods of overnight wear, their clinical effectiveness for extended periods may be limited to minus powers up to −6.00 diopters. The edge thickness of lens powers made progressively greater than −6.00 diopters reduces the chord diameter of the central (apical) area. The increase in edge thickness means that less oxygen is transmitted to the peripheral areas.[51] For example, a −7.00 diopter U3 Bausch & Lomb Soflens thickens to over 0.2 mm in the periphery.

The clinical effectiveness of ultrathin low water content soft lenses prescribed for extended wear may therefore be limited to −6.00 diopters. It may be judicious to fit medium and high water contact lenses for extended wear when the lens power is progressively greater than −5.00 diopters. However, constructing the lenses with lenticular carriers whose thickness is less than 0.1 mm may be a way to overcome some of the clinical problems caused by ultrathin soft lenses made in high minus powers and prescribed for extended periods of consecutive overnight wear.

It may be necessary to fit either medium or high water content hydrogel lenses for either daily or extended periods of consecutive overnight wear for the higher minus powers and, of course, for plus powers. It may also be necessary to replace the thin low water content hydrogel lenses with either medium or high water contact lenses for daily wear when a biomicroscope examination of the cornea indicates that the thin lenses do not transmit oxygen in amounts sufficient to maintain a normal physiological state in the cornea.

When soft lenses are removed from the eye, the scleral area and the cornea should be examined with biomicroscopy. Several types of illumination can be used to examine the sclera. Among them are diffuse illumination, low and high magnification; direct illumination, broad and medium beam, low and high magnification; and retro-illumination, low and high magnification. The examination can be made with white light and a cobalt blue filter in conjunction with a yellow photographic filter when the eye is stained with fluorescein. The red-free filter can be used with all of these types of illumination to examine the conjunctival and scleral vessels on the scleral surface and at the limbus.

To examine the cornea, the following can be used: sclerotic scatter, low magnification; diffuse illumination, low and high magnification; direct illumination, broad, medium, and narrow beams, low and high magnification; retro-illumination, low and high magnification; indirect illumination, low and high magnification, and specular reflection, low and high magnification. The examination can be made with white light, the cobalt blue filter in conjunction with a yellow photographic filter when the eye is stained with fluorescein, and the red-free filter.

Although fluorescein is not generally used to assess and evaluate a soft lens fit on the eye, it will enhance a biomicroscope examination if it is used to stain the eye when the lenses are removed.

Some practitioners use large molecule fluorescein because it will not penetrate the lens material; it may be preferable, however, to use small molecule fluorescein to stain the eye when the lens is removed because its fluorescent quality and relatively longer service life make it easier to study the characteristics of a lens-cornea fit.

As for the method of staining the cornea, almost all contact lens practitioners use fluoristrips. However, Korb and Herman[52] describe how they use 2 percent liquid fluorescein for more than one instillation at a time, sequentially administering it for 30 minutes before examining the cornea with the slit lamp. Their results imply that one instillation of a drop of fluorescein made with a fluoristrip will not furnish the information about intensity and degree of corneal epithelial staining that they found when using the 2 percent liquid fluorescein.

However, the 2 percent liquid fluorescein contains thimerosal as a preservative, and there have been several bad experiences with contact lens solutions that contain this preservative.[53] Consequently, pharmaceutical manufacturers have replaced the thimerosal in their contact lens solutions.

Korb and Herman's concept about the occasional need for more than one instillation of fluorescein is a good one. For example, the initial instillation of fluorescein may stimulate tearing, and the increase in tear volumes may cause some of the dye to wash away before it can stain the cornea effectively. Therefore, making two or three instillations of fluorescein may be helpful in exposing corneal epithelial surface defects much faster than with other methods.

A sequential biomicroscope examination of the eye made when a hydrogel lens is removed should begin with an examination of the temporal and nasal scleral areas to see if the peripheral fit has become too secure. Next, the cornea should be examined for epithelial surface changes, edema, and vascular changes. Finally, the upper lid should be everted and the tarsal conjunctiva should be examined for giant papillary conjunctivitis.[54]

A careful biomicroscope examination of a soft lens fit on the eye will furnish clues as to the type of corneal changes one might expect to find when the lens is removed. Furthermore, some corneal changes induced by cosmetic extended wear may not be found when the lenses are used just for daily wear.

In contact lens practice, a distinctive categorical difference exists between contact lenses prescribed for daily wear and those prescribed for cosmetic extended wear. Although the physical and physiological changes that both modalities induce in the cornea and adnexa are similar, they may occur in different degrees.

Biomicroscope Examination of the Sclera and Cornea

Scleral Examination Procedure

1. Stain the tears with fluorescein.
2. Place the cobalt blue filter in the slit lamp and a yellow photographic filter over the microscope.
3. Use diffuse illumination, low and high magnification, then direct illumination, broad beam, low and high magnification, to examine the scleral area temporally and nasally.
4. Remove the cobalt blue filter and the yellow photographic filter and place the red-free filter in the slit lamp. Repeat the examination procedures to confirm the absence of interference with the conjunctival or scleral vessels.
5. Repeat the examination with white light.

Corneal Examination Procedure

1. Use diffuse illumination, low magnification, to examine the corneal surface for interference with corneal epithelial continuity. There will be corneal epithelial staining in the areas where the epithelial surface has been disturbed by either mechanical or physiological means.
2. With direct illumination, broad and medium beam, low and high magnification, examine the peripheral corneal areas juxtaposed to the limbus. There will be confluent areas of arcuate shaped epithelial staining that will vary in width and intensity when the epithelial surface has been mechanically disturbed by lens movement or when dehydration has changed the lens structurally. Reduce the width of the incident light beam, and examine the disturbed area with direct illumination, narrow beam, low and high magnification, to form a parallelepiped and determine the depth of the disturbance.
3. Change the incident light beam so that it is at an oblique angle (from 25° to 45°) and examine the corneal-limbal junction with retro-illumination, low and high magnification. Examine the limbal area for its vascular structure and possible vascular changes. A careful biomicroscope examination of the vessels in the limbal area should give particular attention to vessels that extend from the scleral area onto the peripheral corneal areas.
4. Focus the microscope on the central corneal area, open the slit, and examine the central corneal area over the pupil with

diffuse illumination, low and high magnification. There may be scattered epithelial punctates when there is also peripheral corneal staining. Narrow the width of the incident light beam to form direct illumination, medium beam, low magnification, to examine the pupillary area.

5. Continue the examination using direct illumination, medium beam, low and high magnification. Move the slit lamp closer to the patient's eye and observe the appearance of the cornea in the illuminated area. Corneal edema will have a gray-white, slightly opaque appearance; it will resemble a ground-glass or scratched surface. This examination procedure will also expose thin, vertical linear formations—cornea striae.

6. Open the slit lamp width to about 2 mm and focus the microscope on the nasal portion of the iris. With the joy stick, move the microscope slowly away from the iris and toward the examiner so that the iris becomes blurred as the microscope is focused in the stromal area. Change the angle of the incident light beam by moving the light slowly from side to side while simultaneously moving the microscope closer to the examiner's eyes. This procedure is designed to expose epithelial microcystic formations and vacuoles in the corneal stroma and epithelial areas. It may be necessary to constantly change the angle of the incident light so that it will become very oblique and create the angle necessary for oblique retro-illumination, the type of illumination that is required to observe this clinical condition.

7. Use direct illumination, medium beam, low and high magnification, to examine the posterior corneal area at Descemet's membrane for folds.

8. Examine the corneal endothelium with specular reflection, low and high magnification, for its structure (for example, endothelial blebs). The areas exposed by conventional biomicroscopy are very small, and it is impossible to examine the corneal endothelium for certain changes (such as shape) as well as one can do it with a specular biomicroscope.

DETECTION AND DIAGNOSIS OF CLINICAL PROBLEMS CAUSED BY HYDROGEL CONTACT LENSES USED FOR DAILY AND EXTENDED WEAR

Many of the clinical problems of hydrogel contact lenses worn for extended periods are caused by the existing definition of this modality. For example, extended wear is not continuous wear. Yet advertising by some companies that manufacture contact lenses for extended wear implies that the lenses can be worn continuously, without removal, for extensive periods. Unfortunately, some practitioners advise their patients along the lines of this advertising message—indicating that the extended wear cycle ends when the patient must remove the lens from the eye for whatever reason during waking hours.

Cosmetic extended wear is not an endurance contest. It is intended to satisfy people's desire for lenses that can be worn during sleep. Hydrogel contact lenses must satisfy daily wear criteria before they are prescribed for extended wear. Furthermore, extended wear encompasses two modalities—daily wear and extended wear. It is logical and practial to instruct patients to continue to manage their lenses during their daily wearing periods just as they did before they began to use them for extended wear. This means that they should remove the lenses during their waking hours, clean them with a surfactant cleaner, rinse them with saline, and then resume wear. This routine does not interrupt the overnight wearing cycle; it is simply a way to help satisfy the criteria for overnight wear. A more appropriate description of cosmetic extended wear would be *extended periods of consecutive overnight wear*.

A hydrogel contact lens covers almost the entire corneal surface. Overall lenses prescribed today are much larger than the corneal diameter, 13.5 mm to 14.8 mm. The water they contain is bound, so oxygen must be dissolved in the lens material and then transmitted to the cornea.

Fatt and Chaston[55] have reported that corneal integrity is maintained only when a sufficient supply of oxygen can diffuse through the lens. They state that the diffusion rate is determined by the position of the lid (open or closed) and by the oxygen transmissibility (Dk/L) of the contact lens. The oxygen transmissibility is in turn fixed by the water content of the lens material and the lens thickness.

Compared to daily wear, some of the ways that using hydrogel lenses for extended periods of consecutive overnight wear may affect the cornea and adnexa are the following: The lens surface spoilage may be more intense; the tarsal conjunctiva may become more irritated, with resultant giant papillary conjunctivitis and physical discomfort; the size and length of existing conjunctival vessels may increase; the vessel sheaths in the peripheral corneal areas may fill with blood; and corneal edema, corneal vacuoles, and epithelial microcystic formations may develop. Increases in the oxygen transmissibility of the material can reduce the degree and severity of clinical problems induced by soft lenses used for either daily or cosmetic extended wear. Regardless of whether soft lenses are used for daily or extended wear, however, they should be removed at regular intervals, and a biomicroscope examination should be made of the cornea to assess and evaluate the fit.

Effects of Lens Dehydration

Andrasko[56] reported that as soft lenses are worn, they dehydrate from their original fully saturated level. The amount and speed of this dehydration are influenced by several factors, including lens thickness, water content, ambient environment, tear characteristics, eyelid position, and blink rate. A reduction in hydration causes the lens fit to become more secure because the base curve becomes steeper.[57] There may also be a change in lens power and a reduction in visual acuity. Nesburn and Maguen[58] have reported finding this change for hydrogel lenses with a water content of 55 percent. It has also been found for some low water content hydrogel materials regardless of the minus power in the lens and regardless of whether the lens is used for daily or extended wear.

Lowther[59] states that physiological problems can be created as lenses dehydrate. Perhaps there is a physical relationship between lens power and edge thickness that, when related to oxygen transmission and larger minus powers, transfers the emphasis from center thickness to average thickness for a more realistic measurement of oxygen transmission. The chord diameter of the central (apical) area of a spherical base curve contact lens becomes smaller when the minus power increases. Also, the edge thickness is not always the same for minus power hydrogel lenses made by different manufacturers.

Biomicroscopy can be used to confirm whether a hydrogel lens has dehydrated after either daily or extended wear. The patient may or may not complain of reduced visual acuity and physical discomfort. The practitioner should first examine the lens on the eye for surface deposits, bubble accumulations under the lens, and lens movement on blinking. Then the lens should be removed, and the scleral area and cornea should be examined.

Procedure for Confirming Dehydration of the Lens

1. Use diffuse illumination, low and high magnification, to examine the lens surface for deposits. There may be one or more scattered mucoid (gel) deposits or a thin proteinaceous film on the lens surface. Also, there may be an accumulation of small bubbles under the lens.
2. Focus the microscope on the scleral area using diffuse illumination, low magnification, white light. Instruct the patient to

blink, and observe the degree of lens movement on blinking. The magnification can be changed from low to high.

3. Reduce the width of the incident light beam and create direct illumination, medium beam, low magnification. Focus the microscope on the lens edge on the sclera, and instruct the patient to blink. An ideal situation is for blinking to displace the lens slightly without displacing either the bulbar conjunctiva or the conjunctival vessels under the lens edge.

4. Remove the contact lens, stain the tears with two or three drops of small or large molecule fluorescein (or the equivalent amount of a fluoristrip), and instruct the patient to blink so that the dye will be distributed over the ocular surface.

5. Place the blue filter and the yellow photographic filter in place. Use diffuse illumination, low and high magnification, to examine the sclera temporally and then nasally. When the contact lens has dehydrated, an impression of the lens will remain on the sclera. There may also be arcuate corneal staining just inside the limbus; this staining is caused by a combination of lens displacement on blinking and a change in the lens material by dehydration. It is not unusual to find an impression of the lens edge on the temporal and nasal scleral areas when the peripheral fit is too secure. A continuous fluorescein stained circular linear formation about 1 mm wide will appear on the sclera where the lens rested (see Figure 5–33). Rarely is there

Figure 5–33. Impression of a soft lens on the sclera when the lens is removed.

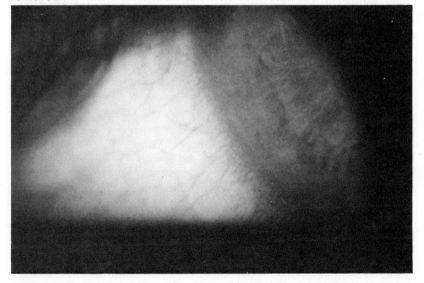

a change in the physical appearance of the scleral or conjunctival vessels in the area where the impression is present.

6. Reduce the width of the incident light beam and examine the
   area further with direct illumination, medium beam, low and
   high magnification.

When blinking displaces not only the soft lens but also the
bulbar conjunctiva and its vessels (for either long-term daily or
extended wear), it indicates a swollen conjunctiva.[60] The swelling
may interfere with the normal exchange of tears and corneal metabolites under a lens. Consequently, the lens should be replaced
with one that has a higher water content and a flatter base curve
so that it will increase peripheral clearance and create a better
lens-cornea fit.

Unlike firm corneal lenses, which may or may not transmit
oxygen, hydrogel contact lens materials can change when they are
worn. They change structurally when they dehydrate, which
changes the lens-cornea fit and causes further corneal changes.

Corneal Edema

Edema is probably the cornea's most universal response to abuse,
whether it is caused by anoxia, osmotic disturbance, trauma, or
disease.[61] Corneal edema may develop among those who use hydrogel contact lenses for either daily wear or extended periods of consecutive overnight wear.

Contact lens practitioners store and use soft contact lenses at
room temperature (20° C) and in an unstressed condition. The information on the lens labels is used to identify and predict the lenses'
clinical performance on the eye. However, when a lens is placed
on the eye, the temperature rises to about 35° C and the lens is
bent or draped onto the cornea, which causes the lens to take on
a new set of dimensions. Contact lens practitioners must cope with
the new dimensions in ways that will assure the continuance of
the normal physiological state of the cornea whether the lenses
are used for daily wear or for extended periods of consecutive overnight wear. A soft lens must fit properly and must correct vision
to stable, normal levels. Thus the values for the lens base curve
and power on the eye are the important ones.

Although a soft lens base curve may change when the lens is
worn, it should always allow blinking to displace the lens slightly
but without distortion and should allow tear fluid to circulate easily
underneath the lens. Chaston and Fatt[62] comment that the tear
fluid must circulate under a soft lens. However, they consider the
fluid circulation as stirring, not as mixing with external tears caused

by blinking. They also state that a problem with some very thin soft lenses fitted for extended wear is that the lens thinness, although an asset for oxygen transmissibility, becomes a liability when the lens clings so tightly to the cornea that it immobilizes the tear film under the lens. Every blink then pushes the lens toward the corneal surface until there is an irreversible thin tear film about 1 micron thick. The change in the thickness of the tear layer will cause corneal swelling. The amount of swelling induced by the change in thickness will vary; thicker lenses will cause more swelling than will thinner ones. The changes that occur in the tear layer are in the area directly behind the lens and in front of the cornea.

Chaston and Fatt[63] also describe the approximate steepening of the ocular surface radius of a soft lens for the various water contents of hydrophilic contact lenses when room temperature changes to eye temperature:

Water Content (percent)	Approximate Steepening (millimeters)
38	0.20
60	0.50
71	0.60
78	0.70

Bibby and Tomlinson[64] report that the basic mechanisms involved in how soft lens materials react when the lenses are worn have not been defined. They have developed a model, supported by clinical evidence, that explains the interrelationship between lens thickness, sagittal depth, and diameter. Hydrogel lenses flex when they are worn, which increases the sagittal depth. The amount of flexure on the eye is one thing; the oxygen tension under the lens is another. The lens may flex, making the peripheral fit more secure and increasing the sagittal depth. Edema occurs only when the oxygen tension on the corneal surface becomes progressively less than 20 mm Hg.

Fatt[65] believes that contact lens practitioners are confused about oxygen transmitted by contact lenses. He adds that some who have written about the subject do not have a clear understanding of the physiochemistry that governs the movement of oxygen from the air through a contact lens (or eyelid in the case of the closed eye) to the cornea. The oxygen permeability of a contact lens is one thing; the amount of oxygen transmitted is another.

A major problem when fitting any contact lens is the lack of knowledge about how much oxygen each patient's cornea requires for satisfactory daily or extended lens wear. The oxygen transmissibility of a lens can be measured to a reliable degree with the polarographic method introduced by Fatt and St. Helen.[66] Their method can be used to determine the amount of oxygen transmitted by a contact lens material, but it cannot predict the performance of a contact lens on the eye. Sarver and colleagues[67] have examined the swelling of the human cornea under soft contact lenses of various oxygen transmissibilities. They consider corneal swelling to be a function of the ratio of oxygen flux into the cornea to the oxygen tension drop across the lens. That is, as the oxygen flux to tension ratio increases, corneal swelling decreases. A successful gas-permeable contact lens material is one for which a small oxygen tension difference across the contact lens drives a large amount of oxygen into the cornea so that there will be less swelling. Regardless of whether a contact lens is used for daily wear or for extended periods of consecutive overnight wear, the lens material can be judged with regard to the corneal swelling it will cause if the oxygen transmitted by the lens is as stated by the manufacturer and remains that way over the life of the lens.

Corneal edema induced by either hydrogel lenses or firm corneal lenses is due mainly to hypoxia.[68] When hydrogel lenses induce corneal edema, there is a loss of corneal transparency and a decrease in visual acuity; also, the epithelium is no longer a barrier to water. The corneal edema can range from mild to severe, with the epithelium abrading if it is severe. The lens must satisfy the prerequisites of a good lens-cornea fit. That is, the material must not dehydrate to a degree that it changes the fit. In addition, the normal tear constituents must be preserved.

In those who wear soft lenses, the edema is uniformly spread across the cornea.[69] Soft lenses do not create the strong physical bearing forces on the cornea that firm corneal lenses do, so there is an absence of central corneal clouding in the apical area. The corneal edema caused by hydrogel contact lenses has no definable border unless it is very severe.

Brandreth[70] described three slit lamp techniques that can be used to detect the presence of minute amounts of edema. The examination is made as soon as the lens has been removed.

Direct Illumination Technique

1. Position the slit lamp at a 45° angle to the microscope, and use direct illumination, narrow beam, high magnification, to create a parallelepiped.

2. Observe a small corneal area directly in line with the pupil edge.
3. Using the joy stick, make a fine focusing adjustment to disclose the minute cellular pattern of the edema.

Indirect Illumination Technique

1. Position the slit lamp at an oblique angle to the microscope, about 45°.
2. Direct the incident light through the pupil to the crystalline lens. The light will create a pale gray background.
3. Vary the angle and width of the light beam to change the intensity of the light reflected from the lens so that the cornea can be examined in retro-illumination.
4. Focus the microscope on the cornea.
5. Watch for a cellular pattern to appear in the corneal area in front of the bright reflex; it will be caused by corneal edema.

Light Reflected from the Retina Technique

1. Position the slit lamp and the microscope in the same plane so that the angle between them is set at or near 0°.
2. Direct the incident light beam through the pupil to create a red-orange retinal reflex in the pupil. Vary the width of the incident light beam to furnish the brightest orange reflex.
3. Focus the microscope on the cornea.
4. Use high magnification to constantly monitor the sharpness of the edges of the light beam passing through the cornea. Edema will cause distortions in the light pattern.

It may be difficult to detect corneal edema with conventional biomicroscopy unless the edema is somewhat advanced. There are usually other corneal changes, however, that make one aware of the possibility of corneal swelling.

A somewhat advanced state of corneal edema can be detected with conventional biomicroscopy. The edematous cornea has a gray-white appearance over the pupil when it is observed with direct illumination, broad and medium beam, low and high magnification, white light (see Figure 5–34). The affected area resembles a ground glass surface.

A biomicroscope examination of a soft lens on the eye will alert a practitioner as to the type or degree of corneal change to expect when the lens is removed. To enhance the biomicroscope examina-

Figure 5–34. Corneal edema.

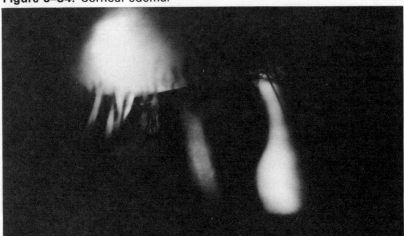

tion of the eye and adnexa, the eye can be stained with fluorescein
as soon as the soft lens is removed. Using fluorescein to stain the
eye after the soft lens was removed, Kline, DeLuca, and Fishberg[71]
found various types of corneal staining. They classified them as
mechanical stains, arcuate stains, pitting stains, inferior closure
stains, and chemical irritation resulting in corneal epithelial stains.

Mechanical stains may be due to improper lens design, faulty
manufacture of the lens, a damaged lens surface, coating of the
lens, or foreign bodies in the lens. Mechanical problems cause an
epithelial breakdown and resulting stain along with the corneal
edema. This staining is usually central and light punctate in appearance. It is believed to be caused by tight fitting, low water content,
thick hydrogel lens. Corneal changes can also be induced mechanically by lens displacement on blinking, poor lens wetting, and corneal drying in an epithelial area, with resultant epithelial dessication.

Arcuate stains are curved in shape, superficial, peripherally
located, and either light, moderate or heavy. The possible causes
are mechanical chafing by the lens edge in the bevel area and desiccation from lid standoff in the area adjacent to the lens edge.

Pitting stains are concentrated punctate stains that may coalesce and deepen into branching patterns with a white pitted appearance. They are located in the superior corneal quadrants. Their
cause is not known, but it has been thought to be related to impaired
corneal metabolism in localized areas under a lens. Another possible
cause of epithelial indentations and resultant pitting stains are
the stagnant bubbles that form under a soft lens that is securely

fitted. The bubbles seem to be water vacuoles and epithelial microcystic formations; they are caused by corneal edema, and they migrate to the surface, where they are held in place under the lens. They are more prevalent among those who use soft lenses for cosmetic extended wear than among those who use them for daily wear.

Inferior closure stains are usually associated with thinner hydrogel lenses. They are located in the lower one-third quadrant of the cornea and result from incomplete closure of the superior lid. Lid pressure causes buckling, which stagnates the tears and leads to corneal disruption.

Chemical irritation resulting in corneal epithelial stains is also known as hypersensitivity to chemical solutions, particularly those containing thimerosal. This irritation creates light punctate stains and dense corneal stains.

Corneal edema may be caused by the displacement of a dehydrated hydrogel lens on blinking, especially when the lens moves over a dry epithelial area.[72] The situation can be exacerbated if the lens edge is poorly finished.

Moderately severe horizontally shaped corneal abrasions are seen with diffuse illumination, low and high magnification, in the superior corneal quadrants (see Figure 5–35). Their appearance suggests that they begin as a series of scattered superficial punctates that coalesce. Their horizontal shape may be caused by forces against the lens created by the upper lid on blinking. Thus a combination of lens movement and the resultant folding of the lens material creates a mechanical irritation to the corneal epithelium. In this situation, the lens should be removed and the patient should

Figure 5–35. Corneal abrasions in the superior corneal quadrants.

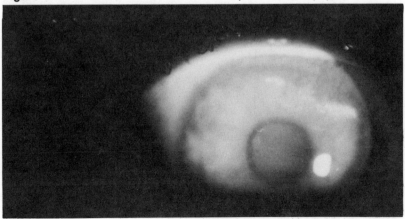

Figure 5–36. Corneal abrasions in the paracentral corneal area.

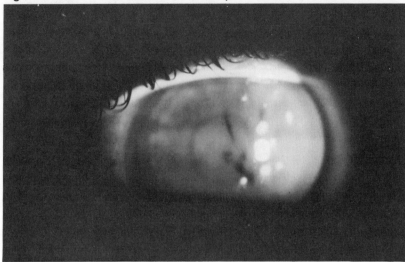

be fitted with a new lens that will have improved centration and show less movement on blinking.

A dehydrated hydrogel lens can cause corneal edema and abrasions in the paracentral corneal area (see Figure 5–36). The abrasions may be scattered from the superior to the inferior corneal quadrants and may vary in size, depth, and severity. Corneal dry spots may appear after blinking. Diffuse illumination, low magnification, should be used to observe the abrasions. To examine their severity, the width of the slit beam should be reduced to form direct illumination, medium and narrow beam, low and high magnification (see Figure 5–37). Severe abrasions that extend into the corneal

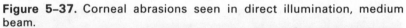

Figure 5–37. Corneal abrasions seen in direct illumination, medium beam.

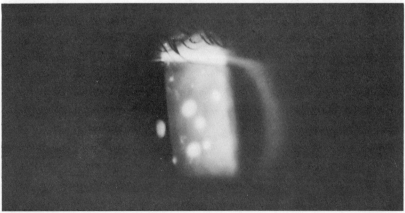

Figure 5–38. Epithelial arcuate staining in the peripheral corneal area.

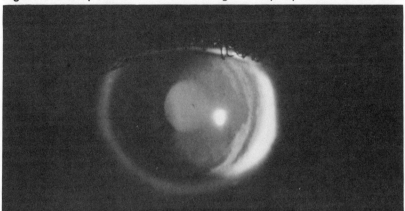

epithelium have definitive outlines and are surrounded by diffuse circular edematous areas. Direct illumination, narrow beam, low and high magnification, should be used to examine the abraided areas for their depth. Retro-illumination will simplify identification of the shapes and outlines of the abrasions.

Corneal arcuate stains in the peripheral corneal areas can be induced mechanically, physiologically, or by a combination of the two. Chronic lens movement on blinking may induce arcuate corneal stains alone or in conjunction with dehydration of the lens material. Also, for some brands of lenses, there is an appreciable increase in edge thickness when minus powers are greater than −5.00 diopters.

Epithelial arcuate stains are found in the peripheral corneal area near the limbus when there is a scleral impression of the lens. They may be located on the peripheral corneal surface near the limbus (see Figure 5–38) or juxtaposed to the limbus (see Figure 5–39). Arcuate peripheral corneal stains are observed with diffuse illumination and direct illumination, broad and medium beam, low and high magnification. Reducing the width of the incident light beam to change to direct illumination, narrow beam, low and high magnification, will create a parallelepiped for examining the depth of the epithelial exfoliation. Usually, this staining causes no pain, discomfort, lens awareness, or change in visual acuity. However, lens wear should be discontinued until the cornea has repaired itself, and refitting should be made with a lens of higher water content and flatter base curve. If the clinical condition has been caused by a high water contact lens material, the refitting should be with the same material but with a flatter base curve. If the high water material already has the flattest base curve available, then the base curve radius should be retained and the refitting

Figure 5–39. Wide band of coalesced corneal epithelial staining.

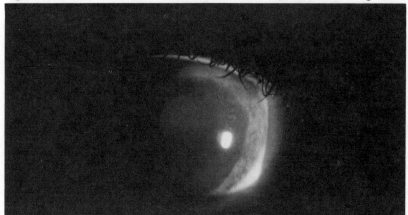

should be with a new lens of the same brand or with a high water contact lens material of another manufacturer.

Bergmanson[73] reported that a corneal epithelial cell divides throughout its life, except when it reaches the surface, where it atrophies and dies. Mitotic activity in the corneal epithelium is reduced when the epithelium is subjected to an anoxic situation. A combination of contact lens wear and corneal hypoxia may prevent the epithelium from reproducing at the rate necessary to match the sloughing off of dead cells. Hypoxia is manifested clinically by edema and scattered epithelial erosion, sometimes termed corneal stippling. The stippling can be explained by the net loss of random squamous epithelial cells. Water gains entrance to the epithelium and causes edema because the intracellular fluid barriers (known as zonulae occludentes) are present in the squamous cells that are shed.

Contact lens wear may inhibit metabolically demanding cell activity and lead to clinical conditions such as corneal stippling and epithelial edema. Dehydration and adherence of the lens to the corneal surface may cause corneal epithelial staining. The staining may interfere with tear circulation and cause corneal metabolites to be retained under the lens, thereby inducing corneal edema. Scleral impressions and diffuse corneal epithelial staining can be observed with diffuse illumination and direct illumination, broad and medium beam, low and high magnification (see Figure 5–40). The dye is absent from the corneal surface in several scattered areas among the diffuse epithelial stains.

Corneal edema is shown to exist in the apical area when an accumulation of scattered epithelial punctates over the pupil is stained with fluorescein (see Figure 5–41). The larger circular cor-

Figure 5–40. Scleral impression and diffuse corneal epithelial staining caused by dehydration of a soft lens and adherence of the lens to the corneal surface.

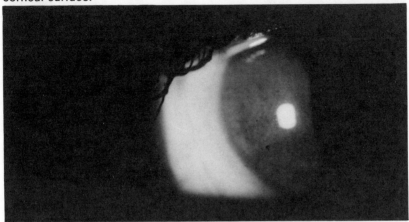

neal punctates may be a form of epithelial pitting caused by an accumulation under the lens of stagnant bubbles that indent the epithelial surface.

Scattered epithelial punctates can be found over the pupil, along with one or more deep epithelial abrasions and scattered corneal dry areas (see Figure 5–42). They can be observed with the cobalt blue filter and the yellow photgraphic filter when the eye is stained with fluorescein. They can also be observed in white light when the filters are removed. Direct illumination, broad and medium beam, low and high magnification, is used to detect and observe the corneal interference. The width of the incident light beam can be reduced to form direct illumination, narrow beam,

Figure 5–41. Edema and scattered epithelial punctates over the pupil.

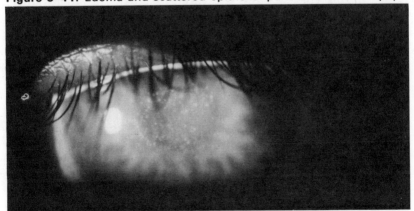

Figure 5–42. Scattered corneal epithelial punctates and deep epithelial abrasions.

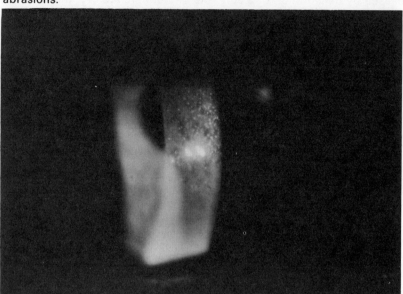

low and high magnification, to determine the depth of the epithelial lesions. Soft lens wear should be discontinued, and the patient should be refitted when the cornea has repaired itself. For this clinical situation and others that are obviously related to corneal edema, a goood fit may become a poor one when the material dehydrates. Therefore, it may be judicious to duplicate the existing lens parameters in a new lens that has a higher water content and a flatter base curve in anticipation of further corneal changes if dehydration recurs.

A pitting corneal stain is created by stagnant bubbles under a soft lens; the severity is limited to the quantity and size of the bubbles and the time they are in position. It is a clinical situation that is associated more with extended periods of consecutive overnight wear than with daily wear. This type of corneal stain has a circular design and may appear in clusters. Pitting stains are observed with direct illumination, broad and medium beam, low and high magnification. The width of the incident light can be reduced to form direct illumination, narrow beam, low and high magnification, so that the depth of the stains can be determined with a parallelepiped.

Corneal striate linear formations[74] are folds in the posterior corneal stroma of hydrogel lens wearers; they are caused by corneal edema and are prominent when corneal edema is pronounced. They may be present in the central or paracentral corneal areas and are usually in the deeper sections of the cornea. They have a gray-white color and good definition and shape, they may be at slightly oblique angles, and they do not have dichotomous formations.

Procedure for Observing Corneal Striate Linear Formations

1. Focus the microscope on the cornea.
2. Position the slit lamp obliquely at about 45° temporally away from the examiner's eyes.
3. Move the microscope closer to the patient's eye while simultaneously changing the angle of the incident light so it will scatter light throughout the cornea.
4. The striate linear formations will show up as one or more gray-white lines in the central or paracentral corneal areas. Focus the microscope on the striae when they show up, and change the angle and width of the incident light for better observation.
5. Generally, use a direct method of illumination (such as direct illumination, medium beam, low and high magnification) during which the width of the incident light can be changed. Narrowing the width of the incident light beam will create direct illumination, narrow beam, low and high magnification, so that the striae can be examined for their density.
6. Move and change the angles of the incident light beam to create retro-illumination, especially when the incident light is reflected from the crystalline lens in the pupillary area. The striae will appear as dark lines when they are observed in retro-illumination in the pupillary area.

Striate linear formations are generally described as having a vertical shape. However, it has been reported that horizontal striae occur before vertical striae, at an earlier stage of corneal swelling.

Zantos reports that corneal striae and folds are best viewed with a 1 mm wide slit and oblique illumination. He adds that at 5 percent corneal edema it is common to have a single central striae, at 10 percent several striae with folding can be expected, and at more than 10 percent endothelial buckling is found in conjunction with folds and striae.

Corneal striate formations are transitory, disappearing when lens wear is discontinued. Furthermore, they often occur in one eye only.

Corneal edema induced by soft lens wear may also cause folds in Descemet's membrane. These folds are observed in direct illumination, medium and narrow beam, low and high magnification. They appear as a series of grayish-white linear formations usually in a vertical arrangement, as if they are parallel, although sometimes they have a radial, or spoke, formation. There is an inherent danger when folds in Descemet's membrane are obviously induced by contact lens wear; a continued distension of the membrane may cause it to rupture.[75] The following remedial changes can be made if folds are found:

1. If the existing lens is made with a standard center thickness, replace it with one that is thinner.
2. Replace a low or medium water content lens with one that has a higher water content.
3. Use a new lens that has a flatter base curve; it is not necessary, however, to change the power for the new lens. It is necessary to wait for the material to equilibrate or for the material and tears to make a pH adjustment. Therefore, a subjective-manifest over refraction should be made when changing lenses to determine if the power in the new lens is satisfactory.
4. If it appears that the lens is too large, use a smaller lens. A combination of a smaller lens and a steeper base curve may be needed when the lens edges stand away from the scleral surface.

Specular reflection, low and high magnification, are used to examine the corneal endothelium. This procedure exposes a small section of the corneal endothelium. Conventional biomicroscopy does not allow judgment of endothelial cell loss or changes in cell shape. These observations require a specular biomicroscope or a biomicroscope with exceptionally high magnification and photographic attachments to augment the existing conventional system.[76]

As for endothelial cell changes induced by contact lens wear, Holden[77] reports on evidence suggesting that hard lenses produce a loss of endothelial cells but extended wear soft lenses produce only a change in shape. Holden[78] also reports endothelial changes that encompass cell density and polymegathism. He considers these changes to be caused by the bleb response, which is itself caused by a lack of oxygen. Woodward,[79] reports that research has shown the endothelial cell count of a soft lens wearer after 5 to 10 years to be equal to that of a 55 to 60 year old person, obviously indicating cell loss.

Endothelial blebs are black areas on the endothelial mosaic that can be caused by various stimuli. Zantos believes that they are physiological.[80] He notes that they are not symptomatic if they appear only during the early stages of contact lens wear.

Corneal infiltrates are indigenous to extended wear contact lenses.[81] They are painful and dictate a need to discontinue contact lens wear until the cornea heals. A distinction can be made between infiltrates that are infectious and those that are sterile. Usually, the corneal infiltrates that develop among some patients who use soft lenses for extended periods of consecutive overnight wear are sterile. They do not stain with fluorescein. The sterile infiltrates slowly regress, with recovery taking two months or longer. It is believed that they represent a hypersensitive reaction to preservatives used in contact lens solutions, such as chlorhexidine and thimerosal. Chlorhexidine may bind to the HEMA; thimerosal, an organic mercury compound, may be absorbed by the HEMA in an amount that is equal to its water content.

Yet another possible cause of corneal infiltrates is papain, which may remain on the lens after being used (in an enzyme cleaner) to clean it. Still other possible causes are corneal anoxia, lens abnormalities, and corneal erosion. The infiltrates should be considered infections unless proved otherwise; usually, they include infectious keratitis and corneal ulcers.

The infiltrative process appears not to be progressive and causes no serious sequelae if it goes untreated. The therapy prescribed is generally topical antibiotics, for example, concomitant topical glucocorticoids. If treatment is not given, the condition may recur. Thus, although the patient can be refitted when the cornea heals, the affected area may reinfiltrate.

Corneal infiltrates are seen in direct illumination, medium beam, low and high magnification, white light, and in retro-illumination, low and high magnification, white light. They have a gray-white color and circular shape and are located in the corneal subepithelial and stromal layers.

Procedure for Observing Corneal Infiltrates

1. Place the slit lamp 45° away from the examiner so that it is temporal to the patient.
2. Focus the microscope on the patient's cornea, using direct illumination, medium beam, low magnification, white light.
3. Scan the cornea by moving the microscope slowly toward the patient's nasal side while simultaneously moving the slit lamp so that the type of illumination is retained.
4. Watch for the corneal infiltrates, which have a gray-white cir-

cular appearance and are scattered throughout the cornea at unequal intervals. The edges of the infiltrates may appear to be spiked so that the infiltrates resemble dirty snowflakes. They are obscured by retro-illumination.

There has been a major change in the methods and solutions for disinfecting soft lenses. Thimerosal has been eliminated as a preservative, and the Septicon system (which uses 3 percent hydrogen peroxide, a catalytic converter, and a 0.9 percent saline solution) is now available for cold disinfection. Septicon is especially suitable for high water content lenses. Therefore, there should be few new occurrences of corneal hypersensitivity caused by preservatives used in solutions for soft lenses.

Cystic formations in the corneal epithelium can be induced by hard or soft contact lenses.[82] Zantos and Holden[83] report finding small, irregularly shaped vesicles in the corneal epithelium after continuous wear of soft lenses for 4 or more weeks. Humphreys and Larke[84] have found microepithelial cysts in the corneas of patients who wore high water content soft lenses for 18 weeks. They terminated contact lens wear even though they did not consider the cysts serious. Although microepithelial cysts may not be serious in themselves, some may progress to subepithelial fibrillar changes, with eventual involvement of Bowman's layer and a reduction in vision.[85]

The epithelial microcystic formations or edema found in those who wear soft lenses cause no pain, discomfort, or reduction in vision. Their presence, however, is due to corneal edema. The formations do not disappear quickly when hydrogel lens wear is discontinued. In fact, their disappearance may take several days or weeks. Wearers of non-gas-permeable hard corneal lenses, on the other hand, usually do experience discomfort, pain, and vision reduction. However, their formations disappear quickly when they stop wearing the hard lenses. Zantos[86] has classified the epithelial cystic formations as epithelial microcysts, epithelial vacuoles, and epithelial bullae.

Epithelial microcysts are minute, irregularly shaped, translucent dots that vary in size between 15 and 50 microns. They seem to originate in the deeper epithelial layers and gradually move anteriorly. In advanced stages, they show fluorescein staining when they reach the epithelial surface. They are usually found in the paraapical corneal sections but may encroach on the peripheral pupillary margins. They may be the result of prolonged corneal hypoxia or mechanical compression by the lens along with negative pressure under the lens. The latter might affect Bowman's layer and disturb the overlying epithelium.

Epithelial vacuoles have an almost perfectly round shape and distinct edges, and they show unreversed illumination. They are of a lower refractive index than the surrounding corneal tissue, and they vary in size between 20 and 50 microns. They usually occur in the paracentral and peripheral corneal areas. Epithelial vacuoles are spheroidal bodies located within the corneal epithelium, but their composition is unknown. They may be either gaseous or fluid in nature. They migrate to the epithelial surface and become trapped under the soft lens. There they can indent the corneal epithelial surface, with resultant epithelial dimpling or fluorescent staining.

Epithelial bullae are probably fluid filled spaces of unknown etiology. They have an oval shape and tend to coalesce into clusters. They seem to occur where there is excessive and persistent stromal edema during contact lens wear. (Zantos has observed them only in aphakic patients.) They appear as flattened, pebblelike formations in the epithelial or subepithelial space.

Zantos[87] reports that an object of higher refractive index than the surrounding tissue will act as a converging lens; the result is a reversed illumination appearance (see Figure 5–43). An object of lower refractive index than the surrounding tissue will act as a diverging refracting lens; the result is an unreversed illumination appearance. Zantos uses marginal retro-illumination to differentiate the three types of epithelial cystic changes from each other and from unrelated corneal conditions of similar appearance. For example, epithelial dimpling (surface depressions caused by air bubbles that form under a soft lens) may resemble epithelial vacuoles when the lens is worn. With the lens off the eye, both conditions will show the unreversed effect when marginal retro-illumination is used; however, the dimples will show indistinct margins and the vacuoles will show distinct margins.

Procedure for Observing Epithelial Cystic Formations

1. Place the slit lamp 45° away from the examiner's eyes.
2. Open the slit width to 1 mm and focus the microscope on the temporal corneal area, using low magnification.
3. Move the microscope slowly from the patient's temporal corneal area to the nasal area while simultaneously changing the position of the incident light beam to retain the oblique angle of incident light. These moves will create several overlap-

Figure 5–43. Reversed and unreversed illumination effects when the slit lamp technique of marginal retro-illumination is used to examine transparent objects in the cornea. Modified from Brown (1971); courtesy of Steve Zantos.

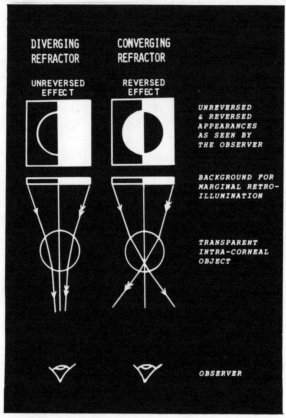

ping types of illumination (direct, indirect, marginal, and proximal).

4. Examine the objects as they appear, using various forms of indirect illumination. Some can be seen in retro-illumination; others can be seen in indirect illumination. Direct illumination will obscure cystic formations and vacuoles (see Figure 5–44).
5. Change to high magnification for further examination and study.

Although Zantos counts the number of epithelial formations, others rely on observation to make their decisions about continued patient management. It may take weeks for the epithelial microcysts and vacuoles to disappear completely, although their number should be reduced soon after lens wear is discontinued.

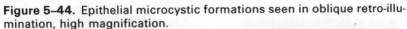

Figure 5–44. Epithelial microcystic formations seen in oblique retro-illumination, high magnification.

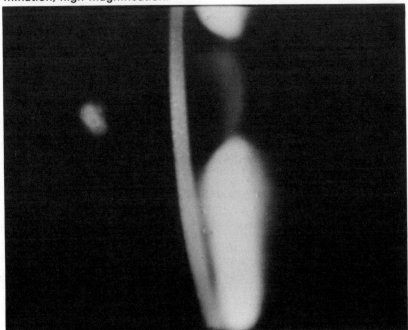

The exact etiology of these disturbances is unknown; however, it is obvious that they are associated with corneal edema. Therefore, practitioners normally instruct their patients either to discontinue wearing the soft lenses or to change from extended wear to daily wear to keep the condition from worsening. Another possibility is to refit the patient with silicone elastomer contact lenses. Because the silicone elastomer lenses transmit almost all of the oxygen in the atmosphere at sea level, the corneal edema will be reduced even if the lenses are used for extended periods of consecutive overnight wear.

Vascular changes induced by soft lens wear develop at the limbal areas. They vary in incidence and severity, are frequently symptomless, and must be regarded as a serious complication of contact lens use.[88] Their incidence and severity are less for soft lenses used for daily wear than for soft lenses used for extended wear. McMonnies[89] has defined the following vascular changes induced by contact lens wear: corneal vascularization and corneal neovascularization. *Corneal vascularization* is new vessel growth in an avascular area. *Corneal neovascularization* is vessel growth in a previously vascularized cornea.

A thorough biomicroscope investigation of the vascular network at the limbal areas should be made prior to fitting soft contact lenses and when exchanging soft lenses used for daily wear for cosmetic extended wear soft lenses. In the latter situation, a description of the corneal vascular state should be noted so that any future changes in the vascular structure can be easily detected. Larke, Humphreys, and Holmes[90] suggest the following descriptive categories:

Eye normal. The majority of the limbal arcades are not filled with whole blood. There are no unlooped arcades or congestion in the perilimbal plexes of vessels.

Limbal congestion. More than half the limbal arcades are filled with whole blood. No unlooped arcades exist, but the vessels are apparently distended.

Apparent early vessel changes. One or more unlooped arcades extend less than 1 mm into the cornea.

Apparent established vessel changes. Vessels extend more than 1 mm into the cornea.

Tomlinson and Soni[91] note the following possible etiological factors for corneal vascular changes induced by soft lens wear: chronic peripheral corneal edema, buildup of anaerobic metabolic by-products, inflammatory chemotactic factors possibly arising from mild disease of the anterior eye, and tight-fitting contact lenses whose base curve and sagittal depth are too steep.

Ruben[92] has stated that the corneal vascular changes induced by soft lens wear have a nonirritant etiology. He adds that they are a compensating mechanism to increase the oxygen supply to an area and remove the by-products of metabolism.

McMonnies, Chapman-Davis, and Holden[93] have described the vascular response to soft lens wear as being due to the filling of pre-existing capillaries rather than to new vessel growth. They also believe that the chronic level of vessel dilation in soft lens wearers is a cause for concern because sustained dilation of the limbal vessels may be a precursor to new vessel growth.

Procedure for Observing Vascular Changes

1. Place the slit lamp 45° away from the examiner and temporal to the patient so that the incident light beam bisects the sclera and cornea.

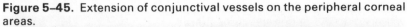

Figure 5–45. Extension of conjunctival vessels on the peripheral corneal areas.

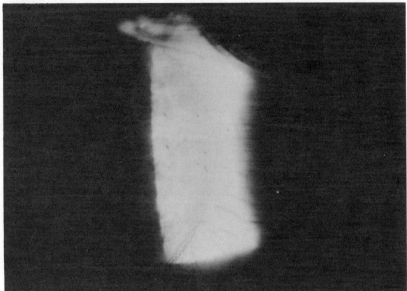

2. Establish direct illumination, broad beam, low magnification, white light, and focus the microscope on the exposed area.
3. Observe the scleral and conjunctival vessels and their relationship to the peripheral corneal areas. The conjunctival vessels may extend over the limbal junction and onto the peripheral corneal area for a short distance. However, they are usually superficial and looped (see Figure 5–45).
4. Reduce the width of the incident light to focus it on the limbal and peripheral corneal areas, and place the red-free filter in the slit lamp (see Figure 5–46).
5. Move the microscope stage and the angle of the incident light so that the incident light is reflected from the pupil. The vessels on the peripheral corneal areas can be observed in retro-illumination (see Figure 5–47). Change the magnification from low to high, and continue the examination with white light. Examine the vessels for the distance of their extension onto the corneal surface, their depth of penetration, and their "loopiness."

McMonnies[94] has used a conventional biomicroscope and high magnification photography to record the characteristics of the superficial peripheral corneal vessels. He comments that the vascular response to contact lens wear can be assessed and described in three

Figure 5–46. Red-free filter used to examine extension of conjunctival vessels onto the peripheral corneal areas.

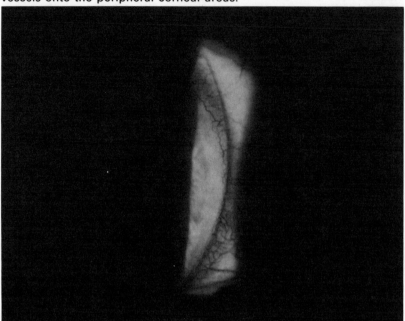

stages: (1) the filling of terminal capillaries that are normally empty, (2) new vessel growth with new vessel spikes extending from existing arcades possibly to form new arcades, and (3) the filling of an established corneal vessel, which may be straight or tortuously curved when growing into the superficial cornea.

New vessels may form in corneal areas that have been damaged by cataract surgery. Although they may be on the epithelial or subepithelial surface, they do not preclude the use of either soft contact lenses or silicone elastomer contact lenses for extended wear.

Nesburn and Maguen[95] have found mostly superficial and inconsequential corneal vascular changes in cosmetic extended wear patients. Superficial vessel growth usually regresses when the lenses are removed, and the patient can be refitted with another soft lens brand or design. However, for deep corneal vascular changes, lens wear is discontinued and topical corticosteroids are prescribed. Although the patient can be refitted when the vessels regress, extended wear must be discontinued if the vessels continue to dilate to the degree that they become a threat to corneal transparency.

A well-managed clinical program for patients who use contact lenses for extended periods of consecutive overnight wear should

Figure 5–47. Vessels on the peripheral corneal areas observed with the red-free filter and retro-illumination, high magnification.

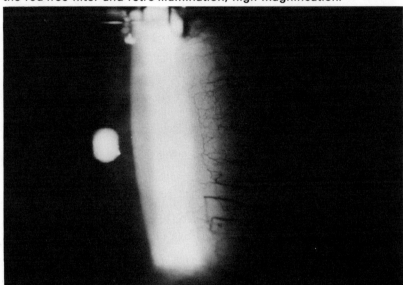

enable practitioners to intercept fitting problems that could cause meaningful corneal vascular changes. Because hydrogel materials can change when they are worn, vascular changes in a noninflamed eye may be a consequence of corneal hypoxia.[96]

Conjunctival Injection

The normally white and clear bulbar conjunctiva can suddenly become injected and red for some who use soft lenses for either daily or extended wear. Practitioners can distinguish between the conjunctival injection that develops as soon as a soft lens is placed on the eye and that which develops after good wearing is established. Conjunctival injection that occurs immediately may be due to a local physical irritation; it will disappear as soon as the lens is removed, cleaned, and replaced on the eye.

Severe and painful bulbar conjunctival irritations develop among those who have been comfortably using soft lenses for either daily or extended wear. *Red eye* is the clinical description for the onset of these irritations.

For extended wear patients, red eye should be regarded as an infection until the possibility is ruled out.[97] If it is not an infection, it may be caused by any of the following etiological factors: toxic reaction to the preservatives in the lens care solutions, the lens fit becoming very secure and metabolic waste materials accumulating under the soft lens, a drop in the tear pH, and poor patient management.[98] The degree of red eye with cosmetic extended wear is somewhat less than that found in the aphakic extended wear patient.

Procedure for Observing Conjunctival Injection

1. Place the slit lamp 45° away from the examiner.
2. Open the slit and direct the incident light temporally to the patient's bulbar conjunctiva to form direct illumination, broad beam, low magnification.
3. Focus the microscope on the temporal bulbar conjunctiva and examine it in white light. Make the incident light beam narrower and wider as needed to enhance the observation. The bulbar conjunctiva will be red and discolored. The conjunctival vessels will be dilated, will move from the fornices toward the limbus, and may encroach on the peripheral corneal areas.
4. Change the angle of the incident light so that it is reflected from the iris, and form retro-illumination, low and high magnification, to examine the vessels on the peripheral corneal areas. The view may be enhanced when the incident light is very oblique.
5. Repeat the examination with the red-free filter in the slit lamp.

Patients with conjunctival injection should be instructed to discontinue wearing the lens if it is still being worn. An investigation should be made to determine the presence or absence of an infection. The injection will clear within 2 or 3 days if the soft lens wear is discontinued and there is no infection. The lens should be replaced with a new one when wearing is to be resumed.

GIANT PAPILLARY CONJUNCTIVITIS (GPC)

Giant papillary conjunctivitis (GPC) is a conjunctival inflammatory condition associated more with soft contact lenses than firm ones[99] and more with extended wear than daily wear. Its incidence is unpredictable, and its exact cause has not been fully established.[100] However, one hypothesis is that it is caused by deposits on the contact lens.[101] Another is that it is associated with allergic reactions. Ruben[102] comments that where allergy is the causative factor, lymphocytes and eosinophiles can be found in the tear fluid or lid scraping.

Vick[103] states that it is common for soft lens wearers to have raised areas or papillae in the area covered by the tarsal plate. The raised areas resemble those of vernal conjunctivitis and may be symptoms of an autoimmune response by the eye to proteins adsorbed on the contact lens surface. The tear fluid proteins coming into contact with the polymer surface may be geometrically (although not structurally) altered. Alterations recognized by the body evoke immunopathological responses; they may be found in some patients who have a predisposition to sensitized reactions.

GPC diminishes wearing time and may preclude the wearing of contact lenses primarily because of the physical discomfort it creates. However, the amount of irritation is related to the severity of the condition, and it affects the comfort of soft lens wearers only when the papillae cover a large area of the tarsal conjunctiva.

Along with physical discomfort, there may be visual acuity variations, bulbar conjunctival injection, mucoid discharge, and photophobia. Discontinuation of soft lens wear is generally used to restore comfort and promote healing. Unfortunately, one cannot predict when the condition will either subside or disappear. New soft lenses should be furnished when the patient is able to resume wearing the lenses.

Allansmith and associates[104] have arbitrarily divided the upper tarsal conjunctiva into descriptive areas and types. A modified version of their division is used to describe the severity of this condition to patients:

Mild. Uniform papillary appearance.

Moderate. Nonuniform papillary appearance.

Severe. Giant papillary appearance.

GPC is an external ocular disorder characterized by a giant papillary response of the upper tarsal conjunctiva.[105] One or more papillae are present on the tarsal conjunctiva; they are situated nasally, temporally, or across the border of the everted lid. The papillae are red-colored elevated areas on the surface, they have various degrees of injection along with a generalized thickening of the conjunctiva, and their overall appearance is that of the cobblestones in the palpebral form of vernal conjunctivitis.

There seems to be no meaningful difference in the relationship of GPC to low water versus high water hydrogel lenses. The incidence of GPC seems greater during the summer than the winter, which may indicate that it is related to the hay fever season or influenced by allergies.

Although other physically irritating lens wearing conditions may develop, GPC is the one to be dreaded because the patient must discontinue wearing the soft lenses immediately and for an unknown and often lengthy period. Furthermore, some who develop GPC can never again wear contact lenses successfully.[106] Many treatments, such as local steroids and cryotherapy, have had only partial success; however, recent studies have demonstrated the efficacy of disodium cromoglyconate (cromolyn sodium) in the treatment of GPC.[107] It seems to help decongest the involved conjunctiva and decrease the prominence of the giant papillae.

Patients have been successfully refitted with silicone elastomer contact lenses (Silsoft and Silsight) once the severity of GPC has decreased; the refittings are done from about 3 to 6 weeks after hydrogel lens wear has been discontinued. The silicone elastomer lenses can be used for cosmetic extended wear without further complications. However, GPC does not disappear completely; only the subjective symptoms of discomfort disappear.

Procedure for Observing GPC

1. Stain the tears with small molecule fluorescein.
2. Evert the upper lid.
3. Place the blue filter in the slit lamp, and attach a yellow photographic filter over the lens at the end of the microscope assembly.
4. Open the slit wide, place the slit lamp at an angle 45° from the examiner, and focus the microscope on the tarsal conjunctiva. Examine the tarsal conjunctiva with diffuse illumination, low and high magnification.
5. Look for the cobblestone appearance of the everted lid (see Figure 5–48). The papillae are elevated, their sizes are unequal, and the dye forms a series of fluorescent channels between them.

It is difficult to control the incidence of GPC. Early diagnosis and treatment are more successful than later diagnosis and treatment.[108] The causative factors of GPC are not completely understood; it appears, however, that the triggering mechanism is mechanical trauma to the upper lid during contact lens wear. Thus it is obvious that the condition will improve when lid trauma is reduced, for example, through discontinuance of contact lens wear.

SUMMARY
Some of the complications of aphakic extended wear may also exist for contact lenses fitted for cosmetic extended wear. However, unlike contact lenses fitted for aphakia, hydrogel contact lenses prescribed

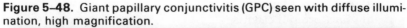

Figure 5–48. Giant papillary conjunctivitis (GPC) seen with diffuse illumination, high magnification.

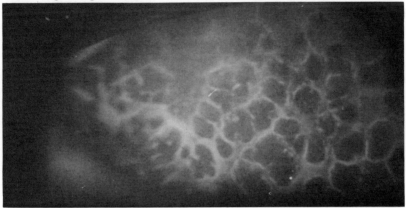

for cosmetic extended wear are for eyes that are nonpathological; some of the lenses are thus very thin and have a water content less than 40 percent.

The incidence and degree of complications caused by the extended wear of hydrogel contact lenses vary. The volume of tear movement under hydrogel lenses is considerably less than it is under hard corneal lenses. Thus we must depend on the lens material to transmit oxygen and satisfy the cornea's demand for it. Furthermore, a hydrogel lens may act as an insulator, raising the temperature of the corneal epithelium and creating a hypoxic environment. A hydrogel lens prescribed for extended wear must satisfy oxygen transmission criteria and must not create a mechanical abrasion to the cornea.

Complications caused by contact lenses prescribed for cosmetic extended wear can be mild, moderate, or severe. They can be classified as:

1. Physical changes to the lenses (mild and moderate).
   (a) Protein and lipid surface deposits.
   (b) Lens splitting.
   (c) Mineralization of the lens.
2. Physiological changes caused by evaporation and dehydration (mild to moderate).
   (a) Corneal steepening and edema.
   (b) Poor vision and discomfort.
   (c) Corneal vascularization.
3. Physiological changes induced by contact lens wear (moderate to severe).

    (a) Acute keratopathy.
    (b) Keratoconjunctivitis.
    (c) Corneal vascularization.
    (d) Diffuse corneal edema.
    (e) Corneal infiltration.
4. Combination of physiological and physical changes (moderate to severe)—giant papillary conjunctivitis.

Physical (structural) and physiological changes induced by evaporation and dehydration cause the lenses to become uncomfortable. They also reduce visual clarity during the late afternoon and early evening.

There is no firm rule that can be used to prescribe or limit extended wear for contact lenses. Theoretically, the extended wearing period should be unlimited as long as the lens surfaces stay clean, wet well, do not interfere with visual clarity and comfort, do not reduce oxygen transmitted to the cornea, and do not interfere with removel of corneal metabolic wastes.

Practitioners should not be reluctant to fit contact lenses for cosmetic extended wear. The use of contact lenses for extended wear is well established and will become increasingly widespread.[109] It behooves practitioners to become familiar with the methods of fitting these lenses and to increase their knowledge of the physicochemical properties of the materials. Only in this way can they prescribe what is best for their patients.

NOTES

1. J. J. Conner, "Ocular Complications of Full Time Daily Soft Lens Wear," *Australian Journal of Optometry* 61 (August 1978): 283–286.

2. G. Andrasko, "Hydrogel Dehydration in Various Environments," *International Contact Lens Clinic* 10 (January–February 1983): 22–28.

3. H. Hamano and H. Kawable, "Variation of Base Curve of Soft Lenses during Wear," *Contacto* 22 (1978): 10–14; C. A. Uniacke et al., "Physiological Tests for New Contact Lens Materials: 1. Quantitative Effects of Selected Oxygen Atmospheres on Glycogen Storage, LDH Concentration and Thickness of the Corneal Epithelium," *American Journal of Optometry* 49 (April 1972): 329–332.

4. Hamano and Kawable, "Variation of Base Curve of Soft Lenses during Wear"; G. Andrasko, "The Amount and Time Course of Soft Contact Lens Dehydration," *American Optometric Association Journal* 53 (1982): 207; L. DeDonato, "Changes in the Hydration of Hydrogel Contact Lenses with Wear," *American Journal of Optometry and Physiological Optics* 59 (1982): 213–214.

5. Andrasko. "Amount and Time Course of Soft Contact Lens Dehydration."

6. M. Sheridan and A. Shakespeare, "Changes in the Dimensions of Soft Contact Lenses during Wear," *Ophthalmic Optician* 21 (August 1, 1981): 502–508.

7. M. W. Ford, *Changes in Hydrophilic Lenses When Placed on the Eye* (paper read at the Joint International Congress of the Contact Lens Society and the National Eye Research Foundation, Montreaux, Switzerland, 1974); M. W. Ford, *Computation of the Back Vertex Powers of Hydrophilic Lenses* (paper read at the Interdisciplinary Conference on Contact Lenses, Department of Ophthalmic Optics and Visual Science, City University, London, England, 1976).

8. R. M. Hill, "In Search of a 'Perfect' Polymer," *Australian Journal of Optometry* 61 (August 1978): 287–289.

9. L. E. Janoff, "The Consequence of Temperature Change on Hydrophilic Lens Base Curve in Gels of Varying Water Content," *International Contact Lens Clinic* 9 (July–August 1982): 228–232; L. E. Janoff and O. H. Dabezies, Jr., "Power Change Induced by Soft Contact Lens Flexure," *Contact Lens Association of Ophthalmologists Journal* 9 (January 1983): 31–32.

10. M. Fox, "More Questions and More Answers," *Optician*, October 1, 1982, pp. p–12.

11. J. Chaston and I. Fatt, "Materials for Contact Lenses and Artifical Eye Symposium," *Optician*, October 1, 1982, pp. 20–23.

12. M. F. Refojo, "The Chemistry of Soft Hydrogel Lens Materials," in *Soft Contact Lenses: Clinical and Applied Technology,* ed, M. Ruben (New York: Wiley, 1978), pp. 19–39.

13. B. J. Tighe and C. O. Ng, "The Mechanical Properties of Contact Lens Materials," *Ophthalmic Optician* 19 (May 26, 1979): 394–402.

14. Ibid.

15. Ibid.

16. R. C. Tripathi and M. Ruben, "Soft Lens Spoilation," in Ruben, *Soft Contact Lenses,* pp. 299–331.

17. Janoff, "Consequence of Temperature Change"; Janoff and Dabezies, "Power Change Induced by Soft Contact Lens Flexure."

18. N. Bier and G. E. Lowther, "Adaptation and After-care of Patients with Flexible Lenses," in *Contact Lens Correction,* ed. N. Bier and G. E. Lowther (London: Butterworth, 1977), pp. 410–424.

19. Ibid.

20. L. Missotten, P. C. Muadgal, and I. Houttequiet, "Surface Deterioration of Soft Contact Lenses," *Contact and Intraocular Lens Medical Journal* 7 (January–March 1981): 27–38.

21. Ibid.; M. Ruben, "Soft Lenses: 1. The Physico-Chemical Characteristics," *Optician*, September 7, 1973, pp. 9–21.

22. Ruben, "Soft Lenses: 1."

23. Missotten, Muadgal, and Hottequiet, "Surface Deterioration"; S. Tsuda, K. Tanaka, and K. Yoshida, "Analysis of Surface Deposits and Effective Countermeasures," *International Contact Lens Clinic* 8 (March–April 1981): 46–52.

24. I. Fatt, "Vision Scientists, Ophthalmologists and Optometrists Meet in Florida," *Optician*, June 4, 1982, pp. 11–16.

25. J. F. Morgan et al., "Blood Constituents and Hydrophilic Lens Coating," *Contact and Intraocular Lens Medical Journal* 3 (October–November 1977).

26. Ibid.

27. Bier and Lowther, "Adaptation and After-care of Patients with Flexible Lenses."

28. R. A. Hathaway and G. E. Lowther, "Factors Influencing the rate of Deposit

Formation on Hydrophilic Lenses," *Australian Journal of Optometry* 61 (March 1978): 92–96.

29. Quoted in Fox, "More Questions and More Answers."

30. Tripathi and Ruben, "Soft Lens Spoilation."

31. Ibid.

32. S. Eriksen, "Prevention of Destructive Deposits with Enzymatic Cleaning," *Journal of the British Contact Lens Association* 4 (January 1981): 36–39.

33. G. L. Feldman, "Contact Lens Materials," *International Ophthalmic Clinics: Complications of Contact Lenses* 21 (Summer 1981): 155–162.

34. Ibid.

35. J. M. Jurkus, T. H. Cedarstaff, and R. S. Nuccio, "Solution Confusion: Photodocumentation of What Can Happen," *International Contact Lens Clinic* 8 (July–August 1981): 47–56.

36. R. M. Hill, "Spoilation and Its Related Implications," *International Contact Lens Clinic* 8 (July–August 1981): 44–46.

37. Uniacke et al., "Physiological Tests for New Contact Lens Materials: 1."

38. M. Ruben, "Fitting Problems," in Ruben, *Soft Contact Lenses.*

39. J. Freiberg, "Deposition of Calcium Carbonate and Calcium Phosphate on Hydrophilic Contact Lenses," *International Contact Lens Clinic* 4 (May–June 1977): 63–70.

40. Hathaway and Lowther, "Factors Influencing the Rate of Deposit Formation on Hydrophilic Lenses.'

41. Fatt, "Vision Scientists, Ophthalmologists and Optometrists Meet in Florida."

42. Andrasko, "Amount and Time Course of Soft Contact Lens Dehydration"; DeDonato, "Changes in Hydration"; Sheridan and Shakespeare, "Changes in Dimensions"; Ford, *Changes in Hydrophilic Lenses;* S. Patel, "Effects of Lens Dehydration on Back Vertex Power, Apical Height and Lens Mass of High Water Content Hydrogel Lenses," *International Contact Lens Clinic* 10 (January–February 1983): 38–42.

43. J. B. Goldberg, "The Practical Application of Biomicroscopy," in *Biomicroscopy for Contact Lens Practice,* ed, J. B. Goldberg (Chicago: Professional Press, 1970), pp. 53–79.

44. G. Young, "A Survey of Ultra-thin Soft Lenses," *Optician,* March 5, 1982, pp. 15–20, 33.

45. B. S. Benjamin and R. M. Hill, "Ultrathins: An Oxygen Update," *Contact Lens Forum* 4 (January 1979): 43–45.

46. R. M. Hill and T. F. Mauger, "Age of the Hyper-thins?" *Contact Lens Forum* 5 (January 1980): 51–53.

47. Refojo, "Chemistry of Soft Hydrogel Lens Materials."

48. W. J. Flynn, T. G. Quinn, and R. M. Hill, "Oxygen Comparison Made Easy," *Contact Lens Forum* 8 (January 1983): 57–58.

49. I. Fatt and R. D. Freeman, "Oxygen Tension Distribution in the Cornea: A Re-examination," *Experimental Eye Research* 18 (1974): 357.

50. R. M. Hill, "Hydrogel Lens Design—The Thick and Thin of It," *Exerta Medica Proceedings of the Second National Symposium of Soft Contact Lenses,* Chicago, Illinois, August 16–17, 1975.

51. Young, "Survey of Ultra-thin Soft lenses."

52. D. R. Korb and J. P. Herman, "Corneal Staining Subsequent to Sequential Fluorescein Instillations," *American Optometric Association Journal* 50 (March 1979): 361–367.

53. Ibid.

54. Ibid.

55. I. Fatt and J. Chaston, "The Cornea's Response to Contact Lenses," *Optician*, March 5, 1982, pp. 27–33.

56. Andrasko, "Hydrogel Dehydration in Various Environments."

57. J. B. Goldberg, "Extended Wear's Low Water Second Generation," *Contact Lens Forum* 7 (October 1981): 55–57.

58. A. B. Nesburn and E. Maguen, "Cosmetic Lenses," *International Ophthalmology Clinics: Complications of Contact Lenses* 21 (Summer 1981): 209–219.

59. G. E. Lowther, "Lens Dehydration: What Are the Problems and Management?" *International Contact Lens Clinic* 10 (January–February 1983): 7

60. H. W. Roth, "The Etiology of Ocular Irritation in Soft Lens Wearers: Distribution in a Large Clinical Sample," *Contact and Intraocular Lens Medical Journal* 4 (April–June 1978): 38–48.

61. S. Mishima, "Corneal Thicknesses," *Survey of Ophthamology* 13 (September 1968): 57–96; R. M. Hill, "Probing the Edema Zone," *International Contact Lens Clinic* 6 (September–October 1979): 29–31.

62. J. Chaston and I. Fatt, "A New Approach to Fitting High Plus Soft Lenses," *Optician*, June 3, 1983, pp. 18–26.

63. Ibid.

64. M. M. Bibby and A. Tomlinson, "A Model to Explain the Effect of Soft Lens Design Specifications on Movement," *American Journal of Optometry and Physiological Optics* 60 (April 1983): 287–291.

65. I. Fatt, "Oxygen Transmissibility as an Index of Soft Lens Performance," *Contact Lens Journal* 11 (March 1983): 6–8, 28.

66. I. Fatt and R. St. Helen, "Oxygen Tension under an Oxygen-Permeable Contact Lens," *American Journal of Optometry* 48 (July 1971): 454–555.

67. M. D. Sarver et al., "Corneal Edema with Hydrogel Lenses and Eye Closure: Effects of Lens Thickness," *American Journal of Optometry and Physiological Optics* 57 (June 1980): 363–366.

68. Nesburn and Maguen, "Cosmetic Lenses."

69. R. B. Mandell, "The 'Tight' Soft Contact Lens," *Contact Lens Forum* 4 (December 1979): 21–32.

70. R. H. Brandreth, "Use of the Slit Lamp Biomicroscope in a Contact Lens Examination," in *Clinical Slit Lamp Biomicroscopy*, ed. R. H. Brandreth (San Leandro, Calif.: Blaco Printers, 1978), pp. 291–328.

71. L. N. Kline and T. J. DeLuca, "Corneal Staining," *International Ophthalmology Clinics: Complications of Contact Lenses* 21 (Summer 1981): 13–26.

72. Andrasko, "Hydrogel Dehydration."

73. J. P. G. Bergmanson, "Corneal Epithelial Mitosis," *Contacto* 25 (September 1981): 19–22.

74. Brandreth, "Use of the Slit Lamp Biomicroscope in a Contact Lens Examination"; M. Ruben, "Complications of Soft Lens Wear," in Ruben, *Soft Contact Lenses*, pp. 293–299; C. Kamiya, "Study of Vertical Striae and Horizontal Striae in Contact Lens

Wearers," *Contacto* 24 (November 1980): 4–9; K. A. Polse, R. B. Mandell, and M. Olson, "Origin of Striate Corneal Lines," *International Contact Lens Clinic* 3 (Fall 1975): 85–88; M. Fox, "Amsterdam Conference—Alive with Controversy," *Optician*, January 7, 1983, pp. 9–11.

75. S. Duke-Elder and A. G. Leigh, "Diseases of the Outer Eye, Part 2," in *System of Ophthalmology*, vol. 8, ed. S. Duke-Elder (St. Louis: C. V. Mosby, 1965), pp. 705–711.

76. Brandreth, "Use of the Slit Lamp Biomicroscope in a Contact Lens Examination."

77. Reported in G. Woodward, "Scottish Contact Lens Society Conference," *Ophthalmic Optician* 21 (May 23, 1981): 365–366; Fox, "Amsterdam Conference."

78. Ibid.

79. G. Woodward, "Scottish Contact Lens Society Conference."

80. S. G. Zantos and B. A. Holden, "Ocular Changes Associated with Continuous Wear of Contact Lenses," *Australian Journal of Optometry* 61 (December 1978): 418–426.

81. G. L. Feldman, "Hydrocurve Soft Contact Lenses for Extended Wear," in *Extended Wear Contact Lenses for Aphakia and Myopia*, ed. J. Hartstein (St. Louis: C. V Mosby, 1982), pp. 103–137; B. J. Mondino and L. R. Groden, "Conjunctival Hyperemia and Corneal Infiltrates with Chemically Disinfected Soft Contact Lenses," *Archives of Ophthalmology* 98 (1980): 1767–1770; P. S. Binder, D. M. Rasmussen, and M. Gordon, "Keratoconjunctivitis and Soft Contact Lens Solutions," *Archives of Ophthalmology* 99 (1981): 87–90.

82. J. A. Humphreys and J. R. Larke, "Micro-epithelial Cysts and Extended Wear," *Journal of the British Contact Lens Association* 3 (October 1980): 138–147; S. G. Zantos, "Cystic Formations in the Corneal Epithelium during Extended Wear of Contact Lenses," *International Contact Lens Clinic* 10 (May–June 1983): 128–147; Zantos and Holden, "Ocular Changes Associated with Continuous Wear of Contact Lenses"; Goldberg, "The Practical Application of Biomicroscopy."

83. Zantos and Holden, "Ocular Changes Associated with Continuous Wear."

84. Humphreys and Lake, "Micro-epithelial Cysts and Extended Wear."

85. Ibid.

86. Zantos, "Cystic Formations."

87. Ibid.

88. M. Ruben, "The Factors Necessary for Constant Wearing Contact Lenses," *Australian Journal of Optometry* 58 (December 1975): 438–442; C. W. McMonnies, A. Chapman-Davis, and B. A. Holden, "The Vascular Response to Contact Lens Wear," *American Journal of Optometry and Physiological Optics* 59 (October 1982): 795–799; J. R. Larke, J. A. Humphreys, and R. Holmes, "Apparent Corneal Neovascularization in Soft Lens Wearers," *Journal of the British Contact Lens Association* 4 (July 1981): 105–107; A. Tomlinson and P. S. Soni, "The Effect of the Design and Fitting of Soft Lenses on Corneal Physiology," *Journal of the British Contact Lens Association* 3 October 1980): 161–167; C. W. McMonnies, "Contact Lens–Induced Corneal Vascularization," *International Contact Lens Clinic* 10 (January–February 1983): 12–21.

89. McMonnies, "Contact Lens–Induced Corneal Vascularization."

90. Larke, Humphreys, and Holmes, "Apparent Corneal Neovascularization."

91. Tomlinson and Soni, "Effect of Design and Fitting of Soft Lenses on Corneal Physiology."

92. Ruben, "Factors Necessary for Constant Wearing Contact Lenses."

93. McMonnies, Chapman-Davis, and Holden, "Vascular Response to Contact Lens Wear."

94. McMonnies, "Contact Lens–Induced Corneal Vascularization."

95. A. B. Nesburn and E. Maguen, "Sauflon Contact Lenses for Extended Wear," in Hartstein, *Extended Wear Contact Lenses for Aphakia and Myopia,* pp. 78–101.

96. J. M. Gordon and D. R. Korb, "The Use of CSI (Crofilcon A) Contact Lenses in Aphakic Extended Wear," in Hartstein, *Extended Wear Contact Lenses for Aphakia and Myopia,* pp. 138–160.

97. Feldman, "Hydrocurve Soft Contact Lenses for Extended Wear."

98. Ibid.; Nesburn and Maguen, "Sauflon Contact Lenses for Extended Wear"; R. G. Lembech and R. H. Keates, "Permalens Extended Wear Contact Lenses," in Hartstein, *Extended Wear Contact Lenses for Aphakia and Myopia,* pp. 44–77.

99. D. R. Korb et al., "Prevalence of Conjunctival Changes in Wearers of Hard Contact Lenses," *American Journal of Ophthalmology* 90 (1980): 336–341; M. R. Allansmith et al., "Giant Papillary Conjunctivitis in Contact Lens Wearers," *American Journal of Ophthalmology* 83 (1977) 697–708; D. R. Korb et al., "Biomicroscopic Appearance of the Conjunctiva in Patients with Papillary Conjunctivitis Associated with Hard Contact Lens Wear," *Ophthalmology* 88 (1981): 1132–1136; G. E. Lowther and J. A. Hilbert, "Deposits on Hydrophilic Lenses: Differential Appearance and Clinical Cases," *American Journal of Optometry and Physiological Optics* 152 (1975): 687–692; S. A. Fowler, J. V. Greiner, and M. R. Allansmith, "Soft Contact Lenses from Patients with Giant Papillary Conjunctivitis," *American Journal of Ophthalmology* 88 (1979): 1056–1061; J. V. Greiner et al., "Mucus Secretory Vesicles in Conjunctival Epithelial Cells of Contact Lens Wearers," *Archives of Ophthalmology* 98 (1980); 1843–1846; J. V. Greiner and M. R. Allansmith, "Effect of Contact Lens Wear on the Conjunctival Mucus System," *Ophthalmology* 88 (1981): 821–832; M. R. Allansmith, R. S. Baird, and J. V. Greiner, "Density of Goblet Cells in Vernal Conjunctivitis and Contact Lens Associated Giant Papillary Conjunctivitis," *Archives of Ophthalmology* 99 (1981): 884–885.

100. A. B. Nesburn and E. Maguen, "Cosmetic Lenses" in *International Ophthalmology Clinics: Complications of Contact Lenses* 21 (Summer 1981): 209–219.

101. Allansmith et al., "Giant Papillary Conjunctivitis."

102. Ruben, "Complications of Soft Lens Wear."

103. J. C. Vick, "High Water Content Contact Lenses for Daily and Extended Wear," *Australian Journal of Optometry* 61 (December 1978): 438–442.

104. Allansmith et al., "Giant Papillary Conjunctivitis."

105. A. H. Malin, "Clinical Demands of Extended Wear," *Contact Lens Forum* 6 (November 1981): 59–71.

106. M. Guillon, "Monaco Meeting on Contact Lenses," *Optician,* 1980, pp. 17, 22.

107. D. M. Meisler et al., "Cromolyn Treatment of Giant Papillary Conjunctivitis," *Archives of Ophthalmology* 100 (October 1982): 1608–1610.

108. J. P. Herman, "Management of Giant Papillary Conjunctivitis," *Collected Letters of the International Correspondence Society of Optometrists* 3 (July–August 1981): 6–7.

109. E. L. Shaw, "A Milestone in Ophthalmology," *Contact and Intraocular Lens Medical Journal* 6 (April–June 1980): 107–108.

Chapter 6

Biomicroscopy for Firm Corneal Lenses

The development of new contact lens materials has changed the characteristics of contact lens practice in recent years. Contemporary practice encompasses a variety of lens forms, designs, and materials.

The first modern change was the development of hydrogel contact lenses. The original Bausch & Lomb Soflens led the way to much thinner hydrogel lenses that also transmit more oxygen. The second major change was the development of gas-permeable firm corneal lens materials such as cellulose acetate butyrate (CAB) and Polycon, the first to be approved by the U.S. Food and Drug Administration. The FDA later approved other silicone organic copolymer gas-permeable firm corneal leans materials, for example, ParaPerm, Optacryl, and the Boston Lens. The third major change was the FDA-approved all-silicone contact lens, Dow Corning Ophthalmics' flexible silicone elastomer lens and its firm hard-resin silicone material.

Although the trend has been to use hydrogel contact lenses as first choice, this does not mean that firm corneal lenses are obsolete. On the contrary, the development and FDA approval of gas-permeable materials for firm corneal lenses has stimulated interest in them.

Hydrogel contact lenses made with a spherical base curve are effective for up to 1.25 diopters of corneal astigmatism and are therefore inherently limited. Consequently, when the corneal astigmatism is progressively greater than 1.25 diopters, a toric hydrogel contact lens is necessary to correct vision to acceptable levels. A hydrogel lens with a spherical base curve and a toric front surface in prism ballast form is also necessary to correct residual astigmatism. However, hydrogel lenses scatter light and flex when they are worn and therefore may not correct such vision to the qualitative levels of firm corneal lenses.

Toric hydrogel lenses seem to work well for either daily or extended wear only when their cylindrical power does not exceed 2.50 diopters. Therefore, it is preferable to use gas-permeable toric or bitoric firm corneal lenses when it is necessary to prescribe more than 2.00 diopters of cylindrical power in hydrogel contact lenses.

Because of the development of gas-permeable contact lens materials, some practitioners forget that millions of people wear firm corneal lenses made of polymethylmethacrylate (PMMA), which has been used successfully for more than 25 years. Furthermore, in many instances where PMMA, a non-gas-permeable material, is blamed for fitting failures, the real problem is poor fitting by practitioners.

When contact lenses are worn, the cornea receives oxygen from one or both of two mechanisms: oxygen diffusion through the material and tear movement and exchange under the lens.[1] The clinical success of PMMA corneal lenses is proof that practitioners have developed fitting methods for contact lens materials that allow oxygen to reach the cornea. Non-gas-permeable corneal lenses can satisfy the need for oxygen when they allow the blinking force to create a satisfactory tear exchange under the lenses and when their designs are compatible with the corneal surface topography.[2]

The biomicroscope techniques and procedures described in this chapter apply to all firm corneal lenses, regardless of whether their materials transmit oxygen. The chapter will also refer occasionally to hydrogel and silicone elastomer contact lenses. However, the biomicroscopy for fitting such lenses for daily and extended wear is discussed in depth elsewhere in the book.

The presence of a contact lens on an eye introduces a new environment in which the eye must function. Because the eye is a dynamic organ influenced by seemingly minute physical and environmental changes and conditions, a close microscopic check is necessary during all phases of contact lens fitting.

An external examination of the eye should be made to determine the existence of any condition that would prevent the wearing of contact lenses; such an examination cannot be considered complete without a thorough biomicroscope examination. The biomicroscope is indispensable in fitting contact lenses and in examining the eye for the presence of minor pathological changes caused by the wearing of contact lenses. It is difficult to evaluate the clinical effectiveness of a contact lens design when the examination is limited to the use of conventional black light and fluorescein.

The biomicroscope should be used routinely, since it furnishes otherwise unavailable information about the contact lens fit. Biomicroscopy should be used in contact lens practice for

1. Examining the eye prior to fitting the lens.
2. Examining a diagnostic control lens fit.

3. Inspecting a finished contact lens.
4. Examining the contact lens–cornea relationship.
5. Examining the eye after removal of the contact lens.

BIOMICROSCOPY PRIOR TO CONTACT LENS FITTING

The eyes should be examined with the biomicroscope before lenses are fitted to determine the advisability of contact lens wear. Although no distinction is usually made between high and low magnification for the various methods of illumination, it is assumed that examiners will select the type of magnification that is best suited for the purpose. Low magnification should be used to establish the appropriate technique and to study a particular corneal area; high magnification should then be used for a more detailed examination of a disturbed area that does not require either a wide field of vision or depth of focus.

For most biomicroscopes, low magnification varies between 8x and 10x and high magnification varies between 16x and 35x; the values are determined by the individual differences of the instruments. On modern biomicroscopes, the magnification can be changed quickly with a dial or a lever. Low magnification furnishes a wider field of vision and a greater depth of focus than does high magnification. The former is recommended for use with sclerotic scatter and diffuse illumination, especially when a cobalt-blue filter is used to examine the characteristics of the dye stained tear layer beneath the contact lens.

Patients should be examined for chronic conjunctivitis, blepharitis, pterygia (especially growths that extend onto the cornea), and any other conditions that might preclude the successful wearing of contact lenses. Contact lenses can be fitted when pterygia have been removed. However, they can recur, and this dictates a need for constant observation.

The appearance of a nevus or of any other pigmented area on the ocular surface should be recorded, and its size, color, and location should be described. Xerotic areas and other degenerative elevated or dry areas on the ocular surface should also be recorded and their location, size, transparency, and vascular characteristics described.

Contact lens fitting is contraindicated when a prefitting biomicroscope examination shows the presence of active corneal pathology other than keratoconus. Contact lenses are frequently the therapy of choice for keratoconus.

Prefitting corneal staining with fluorescein can indicate an early keratitis or ulcer. With biomicroscopy, areas of corneal dystrophy can be detected without fluorescein staining. Dry spots on the cornea are early signs of lacrimal insufficiency, as in the beginning stages of keratoconjunctivitis sicca. Lacrimal insufficiency should be suspected when fluorescein cannot be diluted by the tears.

Placing a Vivitar, Tiffin or Wratten yellow #2 photographic lens filter over the lens at the end of the microscope system will enhance the appearance of the dye patterns or areas that stain with fluorescein when a cobalt-blue filter is used. This is especially helpful when a fluorescein photograph of the anterior segment of the eye is taken.

The presence of old corneal injuries and the characteristics of scleral and limbal vessels should be recorded as part of the prefitting examination, since these findings are of considerable value for later comparison. The following biomicroscope procedures can be used to examine the cornea prior to contact lens fitting. However, small molecule fluorescein should be throroughly flushed from the eye if hydrogel contact lenses are to be placed on the eye during the same office visit. This procedure will prevent discoloration and contamination of the lens by the fluorescein. There is no need for concern when either firm corneal lenses or silicone elastomer contact lenses are being fitted. However, if there are clinical problems when hydrogel lenses are being fitted, small molecule fluorescein can be used to investigate the presence of any ocular surface involvement after the lenses are removed.

Prefitting Examination Procedure

1. Use sclerotic scatter to examine the cornea for normal transparency. Corneal scars (nebulae, maculae, and perforating scars), corneal deposits, and pigmented areas that are exposed by the light scattered throughout the cornea are gray-white in appearance. Corneal dystrophic areas appear as deep, irregular gray-white masses without form.
2. Make a general survey with diffuse illumination, low magnification. Change the angle of incident light repeatedly to allow examination of the sclera and its vessels and the limbal vessels and to obtain information on corneal trasparency without form or detail. The iris appears in detail, and occasionally light reflected from the anterior surface of the crystalline lens can be observed.

It is important to stain the tears with fluorescein and to investigate the characteristics of conjunctival epithelial cells that extend onto the peripheral corneal areas. In this way a distinction can be made between peripheral corneal staining induced by firm contact lens wear and staining that existed prior to contact lens fitting. Diffuse illumination, low or high magnification, and direct illumination, broad and medium beam, and the blue filter are used for this purpose.

The epithelial surface is protected by the precorneal tear film against osmotic damage caused by evaporation. The precorneal tear film is 6 to 20 microns thick and consists of three layers: an anterior oily layer, a middle aqueous layer, and a basal (deep) layer formed by absorbed mucin or mucoid secretion.[3]

The anterior oily lipid layer retards the evaporation of water from the aqueous layer and provides an optically continuous surface for the epithelium. This layer can be ruptured on blinking or by contact lens wear, but recovery is quick.

Tear film stability and good corneal wetting are prerequisites for successful contact lens wear. Fluorescein can be used to stain the tears prior to fitting firm corneal lenses so that corneal wetting characteristics can be seen with the biomicroscope.

Diffuse illumination, low magnification, with the blue filter is used to observe corneal dry spots. A drop of fluorescein is placed on the superior scleral area (bulbar conjunctiva) or on the inferior palpebral conjunctiva, the patient is instructed to blink, and the appearance of the corneal surface between blinks is observed. When the anterior layer of the precorneal fluid is intact, the corneal surface is covered uniformly and without interruption. When the lids are held open or prevented from closing, one or more dark areas will appear in the tear film. These dark areas are dry spots, and they are located in more than one place. However, a local corneal disturbance can be expected in any area where a dry spot is constant.[4]

The timing of the appearance of dry spots can be used to assess corneal wetting and to decide if contact lenses should be prescribed and which material would be compatible. A normal breakup time (BUT) is 15 to 30 seconds. If the BUT is under 10 seconds, contact lenses probably should not be prescribed. To assess corneal wetting:

1. Reduce the width of the beam, and with direct illumination, broad beam, examine the lid margins, eyelashes, masolacrimal ducts, palpebral conjunctiva, and caruncle. Look for nevi, pterygia, and pingueculae.
2. Changing to direct illumination, narrow beam (optical section), traverse the cornea and examine its layers in depth.
3. Use retro-illumination and indirect illumination, low and high magnification, to check for corneal scarring. Also, since contact lens wear affects the limbal vessels, describe any unusual ap-

pearance of the limbal vessels, especially when they encroach on peripheral corneal areas.

4. Using low and high magnification, white light, examine the conjunctival, scleral, and limbal vessels. Repeat the examination with a red-free filter, which makes it easier to distinguish between scleral and conjunctival vessels for size and depth and to examine pigmented, elevated, and xerotic areas on the ocular surface. Also use the red-free filter to observe the extension of limbal vessels onto the peripheral corneal areas.

5. Record all observations in the patient's chart before beginning to fit contact lenses.

Precipitates on the posterior corneal surface often appear. These punctates may be small, circular, bilateral (although one eye may be more greatly affected), and white or brownish-gold. They may be scattered irregularly over the posterior corneal surface or aggregated into the shape of a golden-brown vertical spindle. Although pigment granules are frequently found among the aged, they are not uncommon among younger patients. They may be dystrophic corneal conditions (corneal guttata and Krukenberg's pigment spindle) or familial traits. When, among the aged, they appear as a speckling of dustlike opacities (observed with direct illumination, medium beam, or proximal illumination), presenting a bilateral picture of a floury cornea (cornea farinata), they may be related to glaucoma or Fuchs's dystrophy.[5] When found among younger patients, they are usually a familial trait. Patients who have had posterior corneal precipitates (white or brownish-gold in color) have been fitted with corneal lenses (although the author has had no instances of corneal farinata in his practice). These patients have been strongly motivated to wear contact lenses and have been able to develop long wearing times; however, various forms of corneal interference have been found, among them early development of epithelial denudation and definite prolonged pain after contact lens removal. These symptoms are similar to the symptoms of overwearing of contact lenses even though the wearing time has not exceeded 6 hours.

It has been suggested that although Krukenberg's spindle is inconsequential, it can be associated with pigmentary glaucoma and can be a cause of some corneal lens fitting failures.[6] Dense pigmentation on the endothelial surface may interfere with the mechanism of the endothelial pump if the wearing of non-gas-permeable lenses induces epithelial edema. The presence of a dense Krukenberg's spindle also suggests that the pigment may block glucose flow to the epithelium. (The aqueous humor is the major glucose source for the epithelium.) Therefore, when any of these conditions are found during the prewear corneal examination, the patients should be warned that their corneal state may allow only limited contact lens wear.

BIOMICROSCOPY FOR EFFECTIVE DIAGNOSTIC CONTROL LENS FITTING

It is difficult to fit contact lenses successfully without using diagnostic lenses. Contact lens practitioners usually have a stock of soft lenses, so one of the lenses used for diagnostic purposes may become the prescribed lens. This also occurs when practitioners have corneal lens fitting sets. Even practitioners who do not have fitting sets for soft lenses or firm corneal lenses, however, usually have diagnostic fitting sets.

With trial lens fitting methods, the incidence and degree of early adaptive symptoms are not as great as they are with nontrial lens fitting methods. The biomicroscope should be used to examine the trial lens fit just as it is used to examine regular prescription contact lens fits designed for patients. By using a biomicroscope to examine a trial lens fit, the practitioner is able to assess the lens characteristics and select the proper lens. Biomicroscopy also furnishes information that can be used in speculation about how continued wear of any particular type of lens might create corneal interference. All types of illumination are used for this purpose, but some individual differences are useful in observing and assessing the fit of soft, firm, and silicone elastomer contact lenses.

The initial wearing of a contact lens stimulates tearing and increases the tear volume; the tears affect the lens movement and position and the lens-cornea fit. The tear volume usually increases and then returns to normal levels, the change being related to time and the lens fit. The increase is more pronounced for firm corneal lenses and silicone elastomer contact lenses than for hydrogel contact lenses. Changes in the volume and chemistry of tears may affect the physiochemical properties of hydrogel lenses and induce visual problems. Meaningful increases in tear volumes, created by wearing firm corneal lenses and silicone elastomer contact lenses, may induce corneal epithelial edema. The edema is transitory for wearers of silicone elastomer contact lenses; however, for wearers of non-gas-permeable firm corneal lenses and some gas-permeable firm corneal lenses, a hypoxic environment is created, and the cornea must make a biochemical adjustment to it.

White light is used in conjunction with sclerotic scatter, diffuse illumination, and proximal illumination (low magnification for all) to check a diagnostic lens fit for quality of peripheral clearance, lens position, lens movement or displacement on blinking, and surface wetting characteristics for all materials. Small molecule fluorescein and a blue filter in the slit lamp, augmented by a yellow #2 photographic filter attached to the lens at the end of the microscope system, are used to observe the dye patterns and assess the lens-cornea fit.

The yellow filter can be purchased at any photographic supply store. It is attached to the instrument with transparent tape at the end of the housing that encloses the microscope system. (The photographic filter cannot be used in the Bausch & Lomb Thorpe slit lamp because the telescope tubes are exposed.)

The procedure using white light can also be followed in assessing and evaluating the lens fit when the tears are stained with fluorescein and a blue filter is in place. In addition to the types of illumination just described, direct illumination, medium beam, low and high magnification, is used to traverse the dye stained tear layer so the quality of apical clearance, peripheral clearance, lens surface wetting, and lens position and movement on blinking can be assessed. Practitioners should observe the lens position after blinking, relating it to the approximate amount of displacement on blinking, the loss of position, and then its recovery. For silicone elastomer contact lenses, practitioners need to observe whether the lens fits within the corneal diameter or, if not, how much of it fits on the scleral area and where it is (superior and horizontal scleral bearing); the characteristics of peripheral, apical, and paraapical corneal bearing should also be observed. Diffuse illumination, low magnification, can be used to examine the dye patterns.

In contrast to conventional black-light fluorescein examination, biomicroscopy, with its higher magnification and greater intensity of illumination, allows immediate recognition of the quality of the lens-cornea relationship (see Figure 6–1).

Procedure for Evaluating Firm Corneal Lenses

1. Use the ophthalmometer (keratometer) readings and external ocular and refractive findings as guides for selecting a diagnostic control lens.
2. Place the lens on the eye and allow the tearing to subside.
3. Use sclerotic scatter, low illumination, white light, to examine the lens position before and after blinking and the characteristics of its displacement, or movement, on blinking. When the peripheral clearance is excessive, bubbles will appear under the edges. The bubbles will occur in the central and paracentral zones when the base curve is too flat and the bubbles migrate

Figure 6–1. Diffuse illumination, low magnification, of dye patterns. A blue filter is placed in the slit lamp, and a yellow #2 photographic filter is placed over the microscope housing.

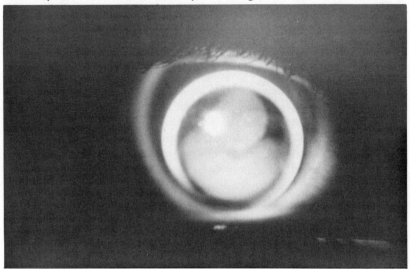

to the central areas from the periphery or when the base curve is too steep and the bubbles are trapped in the central area. When the base curve is too flat, the bubbles frequently move in several directions on blinking; when it is too steep, the bubbles are not displaced on blinking.

4. Use diffuse illumination, low magnification, white light, to observe the surface wetting characteristics. The tears should keep the surface uniformly wet; there should be no drying. However, if the diagnostic lens has a film on the surface because it needs cleaning, there will be poor surface wetting. Removing the lens and cleaning it will restore its wetting ability.

5. Direct the patient to lower her or his gaze; then gently raise the patients upper lid and place one or two drops of sodium fluorescein from a moistened fluoristrip on the superior scleral area.

6. With a blue filter in place, use sclerotic scatter and diffuse illumination, low magnification, to assess lacrimal circulation beneath the lens. A yellow #2 photographic filter will enhance the appearance of the dye patterns.

7. Using diffuse illumination, low magnification, and direct illumination, medium and narrow beam, at an oblique angle, observe the central dye patterns and the approximate quantitative para-apical bearing.

8. Reduce the width of the light beam to form direct illumination,

narrow beam, and focus the instrument and the incident light on the temporal lens areas. Traverse the plane of the dye stained lacrimal layer and assess the quality of the clearance and bearing areas from peripheral edge to para-apical zone, central areas, and the para-apical and peripheral areas on the nasal side of the lens fit.

Differential Diagnosis of Spherical Base Curve Designs

A biomicroscope evaluation of a contact lens fit should determine (1) the width of the para-apical bearing areas, (2) the apparent circulation of lacrimal fluid beneath the contact lens, and (3) the presence of a continuous circular dye pool around the outer periphery. Although present fitting trends reflect apical clearance philosophies that require overall lens sizes smaller than 9 mm, patient comfort and minimum corneal interference have been achieved with lenses that have a minimal dye clearance pool, narrow para-apical bearing areas, a continuous circular dye pool on the outer periphery, an absence of small bubble accumulations beneath the peripheral areas, and an overall lens size that allows the lens to fit within the corneal diameter (either between the lids or slightly under the upper lid).

Air bubbles of various sizes form under the peripheral curve areas when the peripheral curve or the base curve or both are too flat. The force of the blink creates bubbles of various sizes immediately outside the lens. Some of the smaller bubbles may be retained under the peripheral lens areas; others may flush in and out with the blink. This type of fit indicates a need for steeper peripheral curves, a large optic zone diameter (to increase sagittal depth), or a steeper base curve (see Figure 6–2). Direct illumination, medium or narrow beam, low or high magnification, can be used to traverse the dye stained tear layer and observe the characteristics of a corneal lens fit. Corneal apical bearing appears as a dark section, and there is an absence of dye stained lacrimal fluid.

Pronounced apical bearing allows the blink to displace the lens down and below the inferior linbus in such a way that a large bubble may form in the inferior quadrants. Further blinking may form several small bubbles, any number of which may migrate to the apical area and become trapped. This situation dictates a need for a new lens, one that is designed to increase the sagittal depth. The new lens can be made with a steeper base curve, a larger optic zone diameter, or both. Increasing the sagittal depth frequently requires making a power change.

When the sagittal depth is too great, air bubbles of various sizes form directly under the central lens area, rather than migrat-

Figure 6-2. Air bubbles under a corneal lens in the peripheral areas, observed in retro-illumination, high magnification. The force of the blink has created additional smaller bubbles, which the blinking moves to the apical areas.

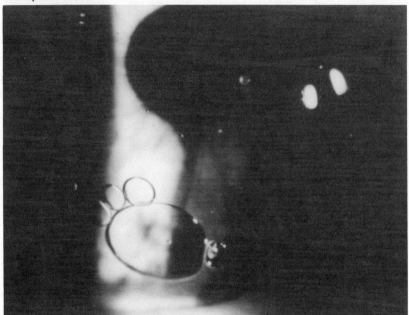

ing from the edge, and cause bubble stasis. The sagittal depth can be reduced by making the base curve flatter, reducing the optic zone diameter, or both, depending on the severity of the problem as shown by biomicroscopy. A judicious move is to select a new lens with a base curve 0.50 diopter (approximately 0.1 mm) flatter (see Figure 6-3).

A corneal lens should show minimal movement or displacement on blinking and should return quickly to a position slightly above the corneal center between blinks. Pronounced or excessive lens movement on blinking will increase lens awareness and induce discomfort, dictating a need to discontinue wear.

It is obvious that when movement is excessive, the lens design variables must be changed to reduce it. However, diagnostic control lens sets use only one size for all the lenses, even though the base curve values are different. Therefore, the only way to learn if increasing the sagittal depth will decrease lens movement without creating focalized para-apical corneal bearing areas or too much apical clearance is to substitute a new lens with a steeper base curve. When a lens with a steeper base curve reduces movement but fits too securely centrally, it is necessary to have a lens made

Figure 6–3. Bubble formations in the apical area observed in indirect illumination, high magnification. The bubbles are stagnant and do not move on blinking.

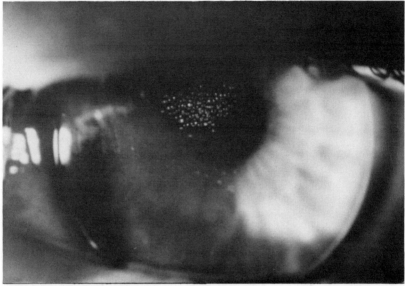

with the original base curve and optic zone diameter values but with the size 0.3 mm larger.

Lens movement may not induce visual distress (such as flare) when the nonoptical peripheral curves do not impinge on the pupil area. However, the pupil will dilate at night during driving, and the prism wedge created by the peripheral curves may cause some degree of visual distress when the lens moves eccentrically on blinking and there is a pronounced background contrast.

Differential Diagnosis of Aspheric Base Curve Designs[7]

The ocular surface of an ellipsoidal corneal lens closely resembles the corneal surface contour; it becomes progressively flatter geometrically from the apex to the periphery, paralleling the anatomical flattening of the cornea's front surface. The shape of the ellipsoidal corneal lens is designated by its eccentricity value. The base curve is actually the magnitude of the ellipsoidal corneal lens, given by its apical radius of curvature.

For an ellipsoidal lens (which is really the end portion of an ellipsoid) the shape, designated by its eccentricity, is independent of the lens chord diameter. For any given eccentricity, a smaller or steeper value for the base curve will result in a lens with a steeper periphery (more downward sloping); the reverse is true for lenses with a larger or flatter base curve. Hence, when overall lens size and eccentricity value are kept constant, changing the magnitude of the ellipse (base curve) will change the characteristics of the peripheral fit and the central fit. For example, corneal bearing in the peripheral areas can be reduced or eliminated when the base curve is made flatter; the lens fit then becomes slightly looser. Making the base curve steeper reduces the amount of edge standoff in the peripheral corneal areas and brings the lens periphery closer to the corneal surface. An existing lens can be modified by decreasing its overall size and replacing the flat bevel (from 0.3 mm to 0.5 mm at the lens edge). This modification changes the characteristics of the edge fit and the location of the bearing areas. Making the eccentricity value larger while maintaining the base curve at a given value will make the peripheral corneal fit looser and the sloping periphery of the lens consequently flatter and less curved.

Using an ellipsoid as an idealized model for the cornea, researchers believe that the average corneal eccentricity value may be either 0.5 or 0.6.[8] Aspheric corneal lenses are currently made with eccentricities from 0.5 to 1.5. Eccentricity values under 0.9 are commonly used for nonpresbyopic wearers; eccentricity values greater than 1 are used for presbyopic wearers (aspheric multifocal corneal lens wearers). When higher eccentricity values are used on normal corneas, base curves may have to be made appreciably steeper than the flatter corneal meridian. A relatively close match of the lens to the cornea, achieved by appropriate base curve and eccentricity values, will minimize both lens movement and lens rocking and will result in good lens centering. Good centering is important in fitting ellipsoidal corneal lenses because the gradual flattening from apex to periphery also changes the optical properties when focus is moved away from the apex of the lens (see Figure 6–4).

Aspheric corneal lenses of any eccentricity value can be used for fitting keratoconus. Steep base curves (for example, steeper than 7 mm) are generally required. Such lenses are deep (having a relatively large vertex or sagittal depth), and their less curved periphery is directed in a downward, long, conelike direction, resembling the surface of the anomalous cornea.

An ellipsoidal base curve has an optic zone diameter that can be measured when the lens is finished with a peripheral curve. (Actually, the optic zone is the chord diameter of the ellipsoidal base curve.) However, when compared with a spherical base curve, changing the value of the optic zone diameter does not change the sagittal depth to the same degree. Unlike spherical base curves, aspheric base curves do not have a straight-line sagittal depth fitting relationship. Making the optic zone diameter of an aspheric base

Figure 6–4. Ellipsoidal (aspheric) gas-permeable corneal lens, seen with diffuse illumination, high magnification, fluorescein, and the blue filter and yellow #2 photographic filter. The progessive flattening of the aspheric base curve from the apex to the periphery makes it easier to fit the lens with a uniform bearing pressure gradient and alignment dye patterns.

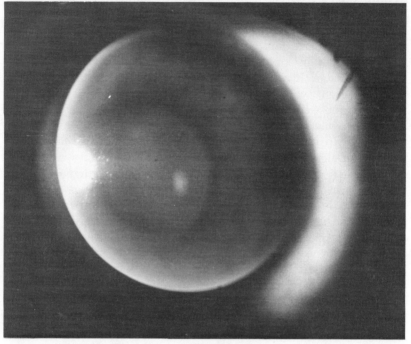

curve smaller is a way to eliminate bearing in the outer peripheral corneal areas and to improve lacrimal interchange.

An aspheric corneal lens fit shows alignment from edge to edge. Because the aspheric lens is flatter than the cornea in its peripheral areas, it is necessary to fit aspheric base curves steeper than the flatter corneal curvature. The amount that the base curve will be made steeper than the flatter corneal curvature is determined by the physical relationship between the eccentricity values of the cornea and the lens and the overall lens size. Thus practitioners must use biomicroscopy to observe the lens-cornea fit when the tears are stained with fluorescein. Aspheric base curves hardly ever fit with apical bearing, unless the fit is for keratoconus. (see Figure 6–5).

Sclerotic scatter, low magnification, is used to observe the lens position and movement. It is normal for the lens to be displaced on blinking. However, lens movement should not exceed 3 mm, and the lens should return quickly to its primary position.

Figure 6-5. Diffuse illumination, low magnification, showing an aspheric gas-permeable corneal lens fit for keratoconus. The dye patterns expose a much larger bearing area over the cone when compared to that of a spherical base curve corneal lens. The aspheric base curve design allows the lens to pull away radially at the periphery.

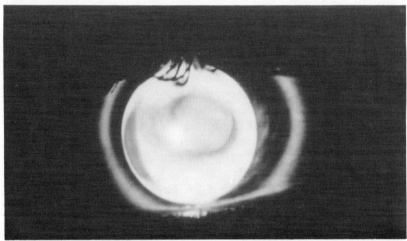

Diffuse illumination and then direct illumination, broad and medium beam, low and high magnification, are used to observe the fitting characteristics of the lens edges. The lens is too loose when there is excessive lens movement and displacement on blinking, especially when the movement creates air bubbles under the edges. Edge lift can be reduced by making the overall lens size smaller (a 0.2 mm size difference will change the sagittal depth 0.05 mm) or by retaining the lens size and making the base curve steeper (0.1 mm, or approximately 0.50 diopter).

Diffuse illumination, low and high magnification, can be used in conjunction with fluorescein, the blue filter, and the yellow #2 photographic filter to assess the lens-cornea fit.

When the base curve is too steep, there will be apical clearance and bearing in the outer peripheral corneal area juxtaposed to the bevel. Reducing the lens size and replacing the bevel curve will eliminate the outer peripheral bearing zone and reduce the sagittal depth, which will also reduce the degree of apical clearance. Apical clearance can be reduced and peripheral bearing can be eliminated by using a new lens with a flatter base curve.

Keeping the overall lens size constant and making the base curve from 0.1 mm to 0.2 mm steeper is a way to eliminate apical bearing. Keeping the base curve constant and enlarging the overall lens size from 0.2 mm to 0.4 mm is a way to increase the sagittal depth and eliminate apical bearing.

Aspheric base curves have an advantage over spherical ones in that they can be fitted with a more uniform pressure gradient on the cornea. The absence of a straight-line sagittal depth (because of the progressive flattening from the center to the edge) eliminates focalized para-apical corneal bearing. This characteristic further reduces the incidence and degree of corneal distortion and resultant corneal astigmatic increases.

Differential Diagnosis of Toric Base Curve Designs

Toric base curve hard corneal lenses are prescribed when the corneal astigmatism is either greater than 2.50 diopters with the material of choice PMMA or greater than 1.50 diopters with the material of choice a silicone organic copolymer. These lenses eliminate corneal distortion and focalized corneal bearing by creating a more uniform bearing-physical fitting relationship in the primary and secondary corneal meridians.

Biomicroscope methods that are used to assess and evaluate spherical or aspheric base curve fits can also be used for toric base curves. Similarly, the modifications for base curve radii, optic zone diameter, and overall lens size parameters that are made to improve the fit of spherical or aspheric corneal lenses are also made for toric base curves.

EXAMINATION OF THE CONTACT LENS–CORNEA RELATIONSHIP

The contact lens–cornea relationship is observed with a biomicroscope, using white light, fluorescein and white light, and fluorescein and a blue filter; this procedure augments the conventional blacklight fluorescein examination techniques. The illumination and magnification provided by the biomicroscope makes this approach superior to the conventional black-light fluorescein technique when the fit of the contact lens is checked for corneal clearance, corneal and limbal bearing ares, and lacrimal interchange.

Procedure for Examining the Contact Lens–Cornea Relationship

1. Use diffuse illumination, low magnification, for a gross inspection of the position and lag of the lenses and, when fluorescein is used, for a gross examination of the dye patterns.
2. Use direct illumination, medium or narrow beam, low and high magnification, to examine the fluorescein picture in cross section.
3. Use all forms of illumination, low and high magnification, to

inspect the cornea for pathological changes. The biomicroscope is not particularly suitable for evaluating the position and lag of contact lenses, since its greater intensity of illumination stimulates lacrimation and often causes the lens to be displaced away from what would otherwise be its regular position when it is worn.

To examine the contact lens on the eye with white light and no fluorescein:

1. Close the slit; then open it slowly to form an optical section, low magnification.
2. Direct the optical section to the patient's temporal scleral area, bring it slowly toward the temporal limbus to establish sclerotic scatter, and examine the lens for fit for lacrimal flow characteristics.
3. Change to diffuse illumination and look for characteristics of lacrimal debris and for any bubbles present beneath the contact lens, including their movement and retention (see Figure 6–6).
4. Form an optical section, low and high magnification, and move

Figure 6–6. Diffuse illumination, high magnification, showing bubble stasis in the apical area under a gas-permeable corneal lens with excessive apical clearance for aphakia. The relationship between the lenticular bowl and the pupil can also be seen. The dark areas are pigment that migrated from the iris to the posterior corneal surface during cataract surgery.

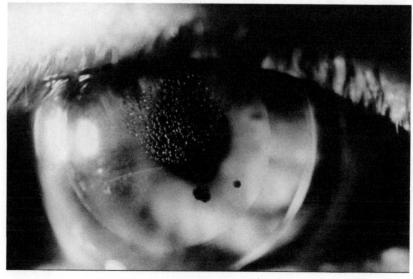

slowly from the temporal toward the nasal areas of the cornea, opening the slit as needed to examine clearance and bearing areas.

5. Use direct illumination, medium beam, and specular reflection, low and high magnification, to examine the front surface of the contact lens for scratches and for wetting characteristics. If the contact angle for wetting is improper, there will be immediate drying of the front surface of the contact lens in the areas where the surface is hydrophobic (see Figure 6–7).

6. Use direct illumination, wide beam, indirect illumination, and specular reflection to examine for lacrimal debris and bubble formations beneath the lens. Change from low to high magnification as required.

7. Focus the microscope on the cornea, and, with direct illumination, traverse the cornea and examine the corneal epithelium.

To examine the contact lens fit with fluorescein:

1. Replace the white light with a cobalt-blue filter.

Figure 6–7. Diffuse illumination, high magnification, showing a scratch on the anterior surface of a firm corneal lens in the central lens area. Specular reflection from the lens surface at 7 o'clock off the pupil exposes poor surface wetting.

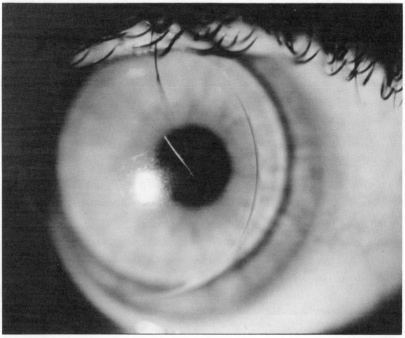

2. With diffuse illumination, low magnification, and a freely opened slit, form a fluorescent glow (similar to that formed using a conventional black-light lamp and fluorescein). Examine for clearance and bearing areas, bubbles, and lacrimal debris. Determine if lacrimal interchange is restricted in the intermediate corneal areas, particularly when an apical clearance fit is prescribed, or in the central corneal areas when it is a flat fit. With diffuse illumination, corneal intermediate zone bearing is exposed, and the approximate width of the bearing area can be estimated so the optic zone diameter can be reduced. Observe the lens position as well as the characteristics of the apical fit so the overall lens size can be modified and the lens base curve can be changed. In time, experience and judicious use of the instrument will overcome interference created by the tearing induced by the biomicroscope.

3. Using direct illumination, narrow beam (optical section), low and high magnification, focus the microscope on the fluorescein stained lacrimal layer. Slowly traverse the cornea from the temporal to the nasal areas to examine for clearance and bearing areas and epithelial disturbances.

The procedures just described can also be followed when white light and fluorescein are used. Direct illumination, narrow beam, forms an optical section through the contact lens and the cornea, allowing the following to be examined in cross section:

1. A small section of the front surface of the contact lens.
2. The contact lens thickness.
3. The fluorescein stained lacrimal line.
4. The gray line of Bowman's layer.
5. The corneal stroma.
6. The gray line of Descemet's membrane.

The fluorescein stained lacrimal line is the brightest of all structures. Clearance areas (especially the outer peripheral corneal areas beneath the lens) have a greater column of fluorescein stained tears; the volume decreases in the bearing areas. The fluorescein pattern observed with this technique has been compared to a wedge of fluid that increases and decreases in volume.

Fluorescein stained lacrimal fluids beneath the central lens portions are indicative of apical clearance, and the quality of central clearance is changed by volume when the base curve of the contact lens and its optic zone diameter are altered. An alignment central dye pattern is simply minimal apical clearance. Apical clearance lenses with small areas of intermediate zone bearing may be clinically acceptable if they do not create corneal interference.

Lacrimal tears and small bubble formations should move freely beneath contact lenses. Cluster areas of epithelial indentations are induced when small, stagnant bubble formations are retained and coalesce. Air bubbles may appear beneath a lens when there is excessive peripheral clearance, usually at the posterior quadrants. A large bubble is flushed under a lens by a blink and will break into smaller bubbles. At first the smaller bubbles are connected, but then they dissociate. Some bubbles are dissipated beneath the lens by further blinking and slight lens movement; others scatter to various apical areas, where they remain to stagnate, indent the epithelium, and induce corneal interference. Apical clearance, apical bearing, para-apical bearing, limbal impingement, and scleral encroachment (or any combination of these elements) are clinical conditions that cause bubble retention beneath corneal lenses.

If the superficial epithelial layers are affected, subjective symptoms of pain and discomfort may be absent when the lenses are worn; however, the patient may report subjective symptoms of clouding or hazy vision. After the lenses are removed, it may be difficult to correct the patient's vision to pre–contact lens wearing levels with any form of conventional spectacle prescription. Sometimes no visual acuity loss occurs while the lenses are worn because the lacrimal layer fills the areas where there are corneal curvature changes and the contact lens furnishes an intact refracting surface. The patient may report visual disturbances after removing the contact lenses, however.

INSPECTION OF A FINISHED CONTACT LENS

The biomicroscope can be used to inspect a contact lens before it is worn and at any time during and after the fitting. The technique, which is the same in all instances, allows the practitioner to recognize lens changes induced by wearing and handling.

To inspect a firm contact lens when it is off the eye, a small piece of black velveteen material should be attached to the headrest of the instrument to form a dark background for contrast. A Q-tip, double-sided tape, or a suction cup can be used as a contact lens holder. Direct illumination, low and high magnification, is used to inspect for scratches at the junctions between all curves (there should be no radial or sponge marks created by peripheral curve forming and polishing) and to inspect the edges for uniform roundness and taper.

When a contact lens is inspected for gross defects, the microscope is focused in front of the piece of material suspended from the headrest (there is no need to focus on the material). A sufficient space must be left between the microscope and the material to allow the lens to be held, moved, and turned during the inspection so individual parts of the lens will remain in focus. Diffuse illumination is used, and the lens is moved or rotated to change the angle of incident light and allow the lens surfaces to be inspected. The polished surfaces should be smooth and consistent, should show no cloudy or gray areas, and should have a high luster. A poorly polished contact lens surface has an appearance similar to that of an orange peel. Burn marks, the result of dry polishing, are slightly dense areas on the contact lens surface.

Specular reflection from the contact lens surface will reveal the normal properties of the plastic material, including weblike areas that should not be mistaken for scratches. (There should be no linear or swirling scratches on the contact lens surfaces, however.) Cleaning or wiping scratches appear as fine, superficial radial marks. They do not affect wearing comfort and are usually present unless the contact lens surfaces are cleaned with air drying methods. The superficial linear scratches that are often found on the contact lens surfaces can be attributed to patient handling and poor contact lens storage methods.

BIOMICROSCOPE EXAMINATION OF THE EYE AFTER LENS REMOVAL

One of the most important applications of biomicroscopy in contact lens fitting is that of checking for minor pathological changes of the cornea or adjacent structures that may result from wearing the lenses. A biomicroscope examination of the eye should be made after the contact lenses are removed, since some of the more subtle conditions can be observed more easily without the lenses.

Patients will probably experience various adaptive problems during the first days of contact lens wear. If symptoms persist beyond their expected duration, they are considered to be abnormal, and corrective procedures must be undertaken. Faulty lens construction and fitting errors require immediate lens modification. Some types of symptoms, however, may not occur until months or even years after contact lenses are fitted.

Because the defensive mechanism of the eye does not warn of the impending danger and because ocular changes may occur without any symptoms,[9] routine examinations are necessary for all contact lens patients, whether or not subjective discomfort is present. Lens modifications should be made as soon as ocular changes are found.

Doggart[10] has compared the cornea to an optical instrument that serves as a window through which rays pass to the media of the eye. He has stated that corneal epithelial lesions may be important even if they do not constitute a threat to the efficiency of the cornea.

Corneal epithelial disturbances can be induced not only by incorrectly fitted lenses but also by misdirected eyelashes, the presence of dust particles or any type of foreign body beneath the contact lens, minor traumatic corneal injuries, and pathogenic organisms, including viruses, directly implanted or derived from adjacent tissues. Disturbances of the corneal epithelium create symptoms of pain, photophobia, excessive lacrimation, and visual impairment.

A thorough biomicroscope corneal examination should be made when contact lenses are removed. It is necessary to use several types of illumination, since each type changes the angles of incident and reflected light and exposes the cornea in a different perspective. Indirect and direct forms of illumination, low magnification, are used for a general survey. A direct form of illumination is used for a detailed study designed to identify and locate corneal disturbances. Indirect forms of illumination are used to examine the areas that surround and are adjacent to the disturbance.

Procedure for Examining the Eye after Lens Removal
The types of illumination described here constitute a suggested procedure; they are not listed in order of importance.

1. Use sclerotic scatter, an indirect form of illumination, for a general survey, without form or detail, to establish the presence of corneal epithelial insult.
2. Use diffuse illumination, a direct form of illumination, for a general survey. It has good exposure for form and definition and exposes the location of corneal damage, particularly when sodium fluorescein is used to stain the lacrimal layer.
3. Use direct illumination, broad and narrow beam, to identify corneal lesions and determine their depth of penetration.
4. Use indirect illumination and retro-illumination to examine the areas that surround and are adjacent to areas of corneal insult to observe definition, translucency, consistency, and pigmentation.

CORNEAL EPITHELIAL CHANGES
Corneal changes induce noninflammatory superficial corneal epithelial changes and secondary bulbar and palpebral conjunctival injection. The limbal capillaries may become engorged and in some instances form pericorneal vascularization when (1) the lens edges

are improperly tapered and designed and are poorly polished, (2) the lens position creates a constant pressure on limbal areas, and (3) the lens is allowed to encroach on the sclera, usually above the superior limbus.

Dixon[11] described the corneal epithelium as being soft, pliable, and easily molded mechanically. The absence of keratinization allows the surface to become indented easily. A large area of corneal epithelium is covered by the contact lens. Because of the characteristics of the epithelium and the lenses, physical and physiological changes induced by the lenses can usually be observed. The changes vary in severity and are classified according to their sequential appearance.

Sodium fluorescein can be used to tint the precorneal film layer and expose surface irregularities and epithelial denudation. The normal epithelium does not stain, but staining may occur when there is an interruption in the continuity of the corneal epithelium. The degree of staining is related to the severity of the damage. Nonstained epithelial edematous areas appear grayish-white when indirect illumination and retro-illumination are used.

At onset, corneal epithelial lesions appear as small areas of edema; they may progress to include areas of epithelial denudation. Almost all of the corneal changes caused by contact lenses are restricted to the corneal epithelium. Damage to Bowman's layer and the stroma is rare, since the corneal involvement is usually superficial. Corneal vascularization is noticeably absent, which indicates that the epithelial changes induced by firm contact lenses are noninflammatory. Corneal vascularization is a major change induced by hydrogel lenses, especially those used for extended wear. (This subject is discussed in depth in chapter 5.) However, corneal changes in firm contact lens wearers can be accepted as local changes that are not caused by general organic disturbances. A staining of the surface corneal epithelium may result from any or several of the following factors:

Design imperfections. Imperfections include improper contact lens design for base curve, optic zone diameter, or peripheral curves; poor edge design and polish; insufficient venting for the intermediate and outer peripheral areas, which interrupts continuous lacrimal interchange and removal of metabolic wastes; imperfect lens surfaces, with scratches, hardened surface emulsions, or foreign material fastened to the lens surface.

Patient errors. Errors include faulty insertion techniques, poor hygiene in handling and storing lenses; and repositioning the contact lens on the cornea from the sclera. The sequential development of corneal epithelial insult caused by poorly fitted contact lenses fit or patient handling is (1) epithelial edema, (2) punctate, (3) stippling, and (4) corneal abrasions and staining.

EPITHELIAL EDEMA

Doggart[12] called epithelial edema in its most delicate form bedewing. Bedewing appears as a disturbed, wavy area resembling ripples on a water surface. It may be local or general and may occur without stromal involvement; it is manifested by the appearance of fine droplets or dewlike changes and appears only in a single plane.[13] It is best observed with retro-illumination, indirect illumination, and sclerotic scatter. At the limbus, in the physiologic state, the droplets are finer, separated, and not easily recognizable. The presence of bedewing may indicate trauma, inflammation, neuropathic disturbance, raised intraocular pressure, or corneal dystrophy. In contact lens practice, it is found to precede the formation of corneal epithelial lesions.

When epithelial edema increases in severity, the surface epithelium is no longer a barrier to water, the epithelial interstices may enlarge, and a corneal lesion develops. The edema disappears quickly when the cause is removed; it worsens when the patient is allowed to wear an improperly designed contact lens. With or without staining, irregular linear forms resembling infiltrates can be observed with retro-illumination, indirect illumination, and sclerotic scatter. When indirect illumination is used and the incident light is placed between 45° and 75° (proximal illumination), the incident light is scattered and the epithelial edematous areas show a dull gray relucent haze that interferes with corneal luster.[14]

When poorly ventilated contact lenses are worn, the epithelial surface of the cornea becomes edematous and cloudy within a few hours. The speed with which the epithelium becomes edematous can be explained by its anatomy and physiology. Any condition that prevents normal physiological passage of fluids or gases through the epithelium causes stasis and resultant epithelial edema.[15] Although the edema tends to be minimal, in unusual cases delayed healing of the epithelium leads to the development of bullous keratopathy.[16]

Epithelial edema that occurs during early contact lens wear may be a normal adaptive condition of the corneal metabolism adjusting with lacrimal interchange to any interference caused by the presence of a foreign body. Boyd[17] reported on 1,000 consecutive new contact lens patients who achieved all-day wear within 2 days. In these patients it was possible to control the lens design variables so that all traces of epithelial edema were absent during this period; the failure rate was 3.1 percent. However, usually the corneal metabolism must adjust to the contact lens through gradual increases in wearing time. Although it is possible for contact lenses to be worn for 8 hours or more initially, they may cause subjective symptoms of pain and discomfort because the corneal metabolism cannot adjust quickly. Although gas-permeable materials transmit oxygen in amounts that should keep the cornea from becoming edematous when they are worn, the development of wearing time for all firm corneal lenses seems to follow the patterns established for non-gas-permeable PMMA corneal lenses.

Individual tolerances for contact lens wear during the fitting period will vary as the cornea makes its physiological adjustment to a hypoxic environment. Practitioners who fit firm corneal lenses made of PMMA generally prescribe a 4-hour continuous wear period to begin with; they suggest that wearing time be increased by 0.5 to 2 hours daily until all-day wearing is achieved.

A quicker schedule for the development of wearing time for gas-permeable firm corneal lenses can be prescribed when tolerance tests are included as part of the fitting regimen and as a way to prescribe personalized wearing schedules for new patients. Thus all-day wearing time for firm corneal lenses can be developed within 1 week.

Epithelial edema may vary from slight during the early adaptive periods to severe when an improperly designed lens is worn for long periods. Intercellular fluid accumulations appear in small, localized areas and spread to larger circumscribed areas, usually over the apical zone, when they are allowed to develop. When there are intracellular disturbances, small vacuoles are observed.

Edema may result from the very nature of the lens-cornea relationship. A securely positioned corneal lens that is not appreciably displaced by a blink may have a high degree of apical clearance and intermediate or para-apical zone bearing. Conversely, a lens that is moved excessively by the blink may have apical bearing and intermediate or para-apical zone clearance. Thus a tight fit may induce physiological corneal changes when it interferes with lacrimal circulation and a loose fit may induce mechanical or traumatic epithelial edema.

When a secure lens fit interferes with corneal physiology, epithelial edema is induced and intercellular staining may occur. The sequential changes in superficial epithelial interference (punctate, then stippling, and finally epithelial denudation) can be observed after lens removal with sclerotic scatter, retro-illumination, indirect illumination, and obliquely angled indirect illumination (proximal illumination), all with low and high magnification. When the pupil is dilated, gross circumscribed edematous areas in the apical zone can be observed with sclerotic scatter, low or high magnification; circumscribed corneal edematous areas in the apical zone can be observed with proximal illumination when the pupil is not dilated.

Retro-illumination and indirect illumination, low and high magnification, can sometimes be used to find an intracellular accumulation of fluid or small vacuoles individually scattered in the deeper epithelial layers. It may be difficult to distinguish a vacuole in the deeper epithelial layers from a small bubble or lacrimal debris present in the lacrimal fluid; however, the diagnosis of vacuoles can be made when, after the patient is instructed to blink, there is no movement or displacement of the formation.

Excessively flat peripheral clearance allows air bubbles to form at the peripheral lens edges. When the bubbles migrate beneath the lens to the para-apical and apical areas, they are broken up into smaller bubbles; these bubbles remain trapped beneath the lens, indenting the epithelial surface and causing epithelial dimpling and edema and intercellular staining. Stagnated small bubbles occur with a secure apical clearance fit as well as with a loose apical bearing fit.

When the deeper epithelial layers are affected, the patient may experience subjective symptoms of pain, discomfort, reduced visual acuity, and visual distress such as clouding and haziness. The edema will lessen and gradually disappear after contact lens wear is discontinued; however, treatment should take account of the fact that the eye is exposed to infection when it is edematous. After the edema has disappeared, lens modifications can be made and the fitting can be resumed.

Keratometric changes greater than 1.50 diopters represent corneal deformation; and if the corneal bending is nonuniform in quality, it must be assumed that corneal edema is present. Although a steeper keratometric finding for the flatter corneal meridian represents a quantitative corneal change, it may be incorrect to assume that this finding is a quantitative measurement of corneal edema induced by contact lens wear without supporting clinical data that describe and correlate changes in the apparent corneal thickness and posterior corneal curvatures. A keratometric change may or may not in itself signify that edema is present; however, the presence of edema indicates that something may be wrong with the fitting situation, and the result may be keratometric, refractive, and biomicroscopic changes. Biomicroscopy is considered the best objective procedure to determine the presence of corneal edema.

In epithelial denudation, fluorescein stains the intercellular spaces surrounding and adjacent to a corneal lesion various hues of green. The superficial layers will show a faint, light stain, and the deeper layers will show a more intense or brighter stain.

Although practitioners seek a lens-cornea fit that satisfies parallel alignment, a firm corneal lens is not fitted in true alignment to the whole surface, particularly when a corneal lens with a spherical base curve is fitted to an aspheric corneal surface. The alignment fit criteria are more easily satisfied when the firm corneal lens is made with an aspheric ocular surface (regardless of its eccentricity value) or a toric ocular surface. Perhaps the reference to parallel alignment deals more realistically with having the lens fit with a uniform pressure gradient so that lacrimal interchange beneath the lens can satisfy the criteria for oxygen supply and removal of metabolic wastes. A firm corneal lens should also fit with some degree of rocking and movement on blinking, so tears will be pumped under the lens.

Intermediate bearing areas are associated with apical clearance. The degree of focalized para-apical corneal bearing is directly related to the degree of apical clearance. Strong focalized para-apical corneal bearing pressures interfere with lacrimal interchange and in time cause corneal edema and distortion. Sometimes the degree of distortion is so severe that it resembles keratoconus.

Corneal epithelial edema develops when the oxygen levels between the contact lens and the cornea drop below the minimum needed at the corneal surface to maintain normal physiology. When there is an inadequate tear exchange behind a corneal lens, water collects in the epithelial layer, the cornea thickens, and the normal corneal transparency is disrupted. Unfortunately, there is usually an absence of pain or discomfort when corneal edema is mild or moderate, so the patient is not always aware of this physiological change.

Central Corneal Clouding

Edema induced by firm corneal lenses is usually located in the central corneal area over the pupil. With biomicroscopy it is seen as a hazy circular or oval-shaped whitish-gray cloudy area over the pupil that becomes denser as the edema becomes more severe and as the edematous area scatters more light. The circular corneal edema is called central corneal clouding (CCC), disciform edema, or gross circumscribed edema.[18]

The appearance of central corneal clouding observed with a biomicroscope is directly related to the severity of corneal edema in the area (see Figures 6-8 and 6-9). It ranges from slight (Grade 1 edema) to significant corneal hazing (Grade 2 edema) to severe

Figure 6–8. Sclerotic scatter, with the edematous area over the pupil weakly illuminated.

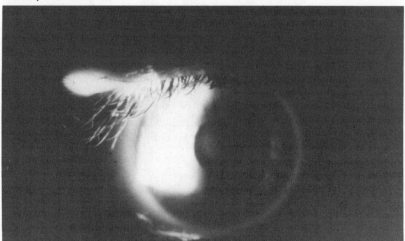

edema with epithelial deposits and punctate epithelial staining (Grade 3 edema). The clouding becomes denser as its severity increases and the permeability or integrity of the cells changes; it can eventually coalesce into a physiological abrasion.

When Grade 2 or Grade 3 edema exists, central corneal clouding can be observed grossly, without sighting through the instrument. The slit lamp can be moved temporally at an oblique angle so that the incident light is scattered in all directions on the cornea. This procedure is necessary when the mirror on the top of the slit lamp cannot be rotated. However, when the mirror can be rotated, the practitioner can sight through the biomicroscope, using sclerotic scatter, low magnification, to detect and observe the central edematous corneal area.

The incident light is from 45° to 65° away from the examiner and is directed to the temporal limbal area. The slit beam width is about 2 mm. The incident light beam can be adjusted so that it is either temporal to the limbal area or partially on the sclera and the peripheral corneal area, bisecting the temporal limbal area.

Procedure for Examining Central Corneal Clouding

1. Place one hand on the slit lamp, using it to control the angle and width of the incident light. Place the other hand on the joy stick, moving it in the direction required to focus on the area to be examined and observed. To observe central corneal

Figure 6-9. Changing the angle of incident light from the limbal area to the cornea, which directs light to the anterior surface of the crystalline lens. The circular gray-white edematous area is better illuminated and more visible in retro-illumination from the crystalline lens surface.

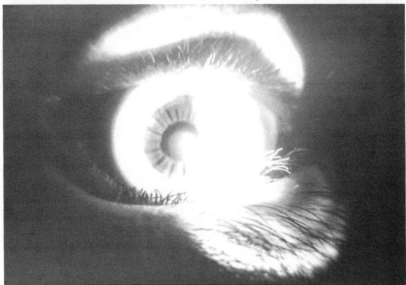

clouding, change the angle of incident light by moving the lamp slowly between 45° and 65° in conjunction with focusing the instrument on the central corneal area.

2. Change from sclerotic scatter to indirect illumination, low magnification, by changing the direction of incident light so that it is now on the iris at an angle that will expose the central edematous corneal area. Focus the microscope on the iris and slowly move the instrument closer to yourself while retaining indirect illumination. During this procedure, look for small droplets that may form in the deeper epithelium or anterior stroma when the edema is severe. These droplets are microcystic formations.

3. Although indirect illumination is the method that is first used to detect microcystic formations, they can also be detected by using direct illumination, medium to narrow beam, low or high magnification, when the edema is severe. Use retro-illumination and direct illumination, medium beam, low and high magnification, to examine the area for denseness and for the presence of mycrocystic formations. The formations can be more easily detected by changing the angles of incident light.

4. Observe scattered superficial punctate staining on the surface of the edematous area, when the condition is severe, with direct

illumination, low and high magnification, white light, and then the blue filter.

Central corneal clouding dissipates when the lens is removed and wear is discontinued. Refitting can begin when a later biomicroscope examination and a chronological record of the refractive state confirm that the cornea has recovered.

PUNCTATE AND STIPPLING

A punctate is a small (pinpoint), usually superficial single lesion of the corneal epithelium that may cause pain when it affects the deeper epithelial layers. It often is accompanied by conjunctivitis, photophobia, excessive lacrimation, mild ciliary injection, and edema in the surrounding areas. It occurs when a contact lens interferes with lacrimal interchange; subjective symptoms may not appear for a while. If the condition is not corrected, the punctates increase in size and number and coalesce into large areas of staining. A series of superficial pinpoint epithelial punctates is often termed stippling. Punctates and stippling do not indent the epithelial surface.

A punctate epithelial lesion appears as a grayish-white area with circumscribed edema. Varying degrees of dye retention characterize the surrounding area immediately after 2 or more hours of contact lens wear. The lesion may not create visual disturbance. In cases of keratoconus, the lesion is usually found where a contact lens has been resting constantly against the cone apex (see Figure 6–10).

Sclerotic scatter, diffuse illumination and direct illumination, medium beam, are used to expose and locate punctates. An optical section formed by the narrow beam of direct illumination is used to determine the depth of epithelial penetration; indirect illumination and retro-illumination are used to examine the adjacent corneal areas for epithelial edema.

Contact lens wear should be discontinued until epithelial regeneration has repaired the affected area. Lens modification may then be appropriate.

CORNEAL ABRASIONS AND STAINING

Corneal abrasions from contact lens wear may be caused by mechanical trauma or by an improper lens-cornea relationship; either one may disturb the normal structure of the corneal epithelium and induce physiological epithelial changes such as edema and desquamation or exfoliation. The severity of the epithelial disturbance is directly related to wearing time and the characteristics of the

Figure 6-10. Direct illumination, high magnification, showing scattered punctates.

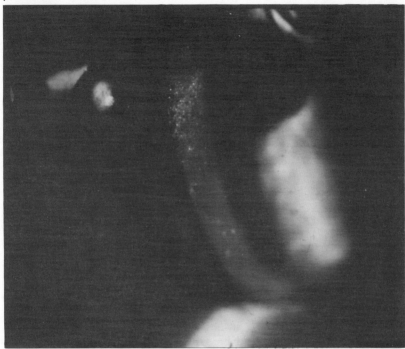

causes. Corneal abrasions may be the result of late diagnosis of edema caused by contact lens wear.

The cornea abrades when trauma causes an interruption or removal of part of the epithelial surface; in contact lens practice, *corneal abrasion* literally means a rubbing off of the epithelial cells. However, the word *erosion* has been used to describe recurrent corneal abrasion. The word *staining* refers to the fact that the corneal tissue is stained by fluorescein that has been instilled into the eye. Therefore, for all practical purposes, erosion, staining, and denudation are all synonymous with abrasion (see Figure 6–11).

An improper lens fit, either flat or steep, creates a faulty lens-cornea relationship. The movement of a flat-fitting lens has a mechanical massaging effect on the epithelium; the movement may become abrasive, and the sharp junctions between posterior surface curves (poorly blended junctions) may induce the epithelium to fold into minute branching furrows so that it wrinkles and gathers at the lens periphery. Using a biomicroscope, low or high magnification, and indirect illumination, proximal illumination or retro-illumination, the practitioner can observe irregular linear staining or small edematous adjacent areas. A flat fit may cause premature

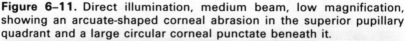

Figure 6–11. Direct illumination, medium beam, low magnification, showing an arcuate-shaped corneal abrasion in the superior pupillary quadrant and a large circular corneal punctate beneath it.

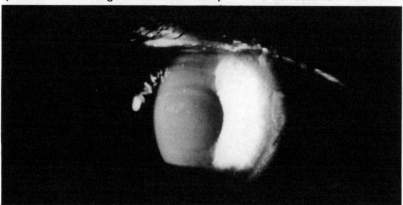

desquamation of the superficial epithelial cells, exposing the immature cells beneath a series of fine spotty lesions scattered over any part of the cornea. Occasionally, when the inside edges of a corneal lens are improperly polished or shaped, lens movement will cause desquamation of the epithelial cells at the peripheral corneal areas, which may stain. When this condition becomes severe, it induces photophobia and lacrimation.

With a steep fit, corneal bearing areas in the para-apical zone may cause corneal deformation or a change in corneal structures; the patient experiences subjective symptoms of burning, stinging, and foggy and hazy vision. Using retro-illumination, indirect illumination, or proximal illumination, low or high magnification, the practitioner can observe superficial epithelial abrasions such as a single punctate, multiple punctates (stippling), epithelial exfoliation or desquamation, intercellular staining, intracellular vacuoles, and epithelial edema. Clinical examination of the corneal lens fit and modification of the lens variables will prevent severe problems. However, when a patient disregards instructions and overwears the lenses, severe epithelial desquamation may result. When steep (tight) corneal lens are overworn, epithelial edema is induced by the lack of corneal exposure to atmospheric oxygen, by a decrease in the hypertonicity of the tears, or by some unknown etiologic factor.[19] Subjective symptoms of pain, lacrimation, photophobia, and decreased vision are experienced, and the discomfort may continue 12 hours or more. Biomicroscopically, there are edema, superficial punctates, and staining; the confluence of affected areas often produces a large area of staining.

Corneal abrasions may recur (recurrent abrasions) when corneal lens wear is resumed before an epithelial disturbance is completely healed. The cornea should be examined with retro-illumination, low or high magnification, for small vesicles (intracellular vacuoles) to make sure that the healing is complete.

Aperture fenestrations were sometimes placed in corneal lenses made of PMMA as a way to dissipate stagnant lacrimal fluid accumulations beneath the apical area. However, the availability of gas-permeable corneal lenses has made this procedure obsolete.

Mechanical epithelial trauma may occur when a patient recenters a corneal lens that has been displaced on the sclera. The resulting irregularly shaped abraded areas are usually superficial and transitory; they can be observed with diffuse illumination, direct illumination, medium beam, and indirect illumination, low and high magnification.

Occasionally, substances such as oils from the fingers, meibomian secretions, or mucous particles may induce mechanical trauma to the epithelial surface when they preclude proper wetting or cleaning and become crusty formations adhering to the posterior lens surface.

Corneal abrasions caused by faulty insertion techniques are crescent-shaped. Those caused by foreign particles such as dust and mascara trapped under the lens appear as swirling, irregular radial lines that may retain fluorescein.

Sclerotic scatter and diffuse illumination are used for a general survey of corneal abrasions. Direct illumination, wide beam, is used to study the superficial epithelium. An optic section, formed by direct illumination, narrow beam, is used to determine its depth. Indirect illumination and retro-illumination are used to examine the surrounding areas for epithelial edema. Both low and high magnification should be used for all types of illumination.

Phosphatase is found in cellular elements of the stroma of the normal cornea. After epithelial abrasion, a strong phosphatase reaction with lymphocytes occurs in the interlamellar spaces immediately underneath the affected area. The lymphocytes quickly increase in number and then gradually decrease as the cornea returns to normal. There is cell migration to cover the injured area, and mitosis reconstitutes the normal number of epithelial cells.

Although recovery from corneal abrasion occurs rapidly after contact lens removal, any abraded surface represents a potentially infectious site, and the need for medical treatment should not be ignored. The patient should not wear the lenses again until epithelial regeneration has repaired the affected areas.

Peripheral Corneal Staining at 3 O'clock and 9 O'clock

The corneal insult induced by firm corneal lens wear is appropriately named peripheral corneal staining at 3 o'clock and 9 o'clock because it is in the horizontal corneal meredian, just inside the limbus and within the palpebral aperture. It may be on both sides of the cornea or only on the nasal or temporal side.

The staining varies in severity from diffuse random punctate dots to concentrated coalesced punctate lesions.[20] This rather unusual type of corneal staining may be caused by desiccation of the corneal epithelium adjacent to the contact lens edge that is the result of insufficient wetting, or drying. Other, related etiological factors are mechanical trauma, inadequate blinking, and a dry corneal surface. Staining at 3 o'clock and 9 o'clock was first noticed in the era when small, thin corneal lenses were fitted within the palpebral aperture between the lids. Little, if any, of this staining occurred during the period when hard corneal lenses were designed according to the contour fitting philosophy.

Contact lens materials have been changed from PMMA to Polycon to Silcon to CAB in the quest for a material with low wetting angles that might reduce or eliminate 3–9 corneal staining. None of these materials caused any change, however. Therefore, perhaps the problem is caused by the drying of the exposed corneal surface that results from inadequate blinking.

To observe 3–9 corneal staining with biomicroscopy, the tears are stained with fluorescein and the staining is examined with direct illumination, medium beam, low and high magnification, white light, and then the blue filter. The area is examined for its shape, size, and extent of penetration onto the corneal surface.

It does not always follow that 3–9 peripheral corneal staining is caused by corneal lens wear. When an examination is made of the eye prior to contact lens fitting, staining the tears with fluorescein and using direct illumination, medium beam, low magnification, and the blue filter to examine the scleral area, the practitioner can sometimes observe that conjunctival epithelial cells have extended onto the peripheral corneal area, resembling 3–9 staining.

In addition to the epithelial disturbances described in this section, there are other clinical conditions precluding good wear. They are related to the environment or to improperly fitted corneal lenses and include epithelial dimpling, foreign bodies embedded in the cornea, changes in corneal curvature and refractive status, and limbal vessel proliferation.

EPITHELIAL DIMPLING

The group of depressed areas, or dimples, that form in the corneal epithelium as a result of the retention of bubbles beneath the contact lenses are known as epithelial dimpling. They appear in clusters in the superior and para-apical corneal zones, are painless, produce no inflammatory reaction, induce ophthalmometer mire distortion, and may cause the patient to experience blurred vision with any form of spectacle prescription from several hours to as much as 2 days after contact lenses are removed. Fluorescein will collect in the depressed areas, but most of it can be flushed out with irrigation fluid. The condition is usually associated with a securely fitting high-riding lens that causes air to stagnate under it. If allowed to persist, the dimpling leads to interference with corneal metabolism and to epithelial edema in the adjacent areas. The condition is also associated with excessively flat peripheral curves that allow air bubbles to form under the peripheral lens areas and migrate to the apical areas, where they stagnate.

Dixon and Lawaczek[21] made an exhaustive study of epithelial dimpling. They reported that the dimples are transient and associated with impaired tear flow under corneal lenses and that the exact mechanism of the formation of the dimples is unknown but they do not appear to be due to a broken epithelial surface.

According to Dickinson,[22] these bubbles are due to corneal asphyxiation. Dixon and Lawaczek,[23] however, believe that the air bubbles do not cause the depressions but instead fill the indented corneal areas after they are formed.

Schapero[24] comments that Dixon and Lawaczek's view might be a definite possibility when the blink moves the corneal lens downward so the lens edges flare away from the cornea and allow air to enter between the lens and cornea. After the blink, when the lens returns to its original upward position, air is sealed in the superior corneal quadrants beneath the lens. According to Schapero, bubble formations seen in steep fits do not appear to be caused in the same manner, since the intermediate (para-apical) ring of touch that surrounds the central stagnant pool tends to prevent air bubbles from passing into this area. Schapero accepts Dickinson's opinion that the bubbles are collections of gaseous metabolic waste products.

Whether or not bubble formations found beneath a corneal lens are air bubbles or gaseous bubbles, blinking seems to create a constant force against stagnant, trapped bubbles so that the epithelium is indented, the interstices enlarge, and small, irregularly shaped corneal abrasions of various sizes are formed in adjacent edematous areas. The severity of the epithelial indentations and their differences in shape and size may be related to the bubble sizes and the force against them; all of these factors seem to be influenced by the length of time that the condition exists.

When an improper contact lens design induces epithelial

edema, the separation of the intercellular spaces becomes greater as the wearing time increases; and when bubbles are retained beneath a corneal lens, they migrate toward the intercellular spaces and fill them. Thus concave epithelial indentations are formed by the lens exerting a constant pressure against the bubbles. When the lens is removed, the corneal epithelial indentations are no longer filled with bubbles and disappear after a few hours. If allowed to remain, the areas may coalesce, cause epithelial erosion, create deeper, more diffuse epithelial abrasions, and produce pain and discomfort.

Low or high magnification, sclerotic scatter, and diffuse illumination and direct illumination, medium beam, are used to expose the dimpling. When the dye is retained, direct illumination, narrow beam, is used to determine the depth of epithelial penetration.

Indirect illumination and retro-illumination are used to examine the adjacent areas for epithelial edema. The corneal areas between the indentations are usually clear, and epithelial dimpling often casts shadows against the iris.

Contact lens wear should be discontinued until the epithelium regenerates and the lens design is modified, if this is appropriate. Such modification facilitates improvement in lacrimal interchange.

FOREIGN BODY LESIONS

Foreign body lesions may result from a chemically active or chemically inert foreign body that has invaded the cornea. It is more common than usual in certain occupational environments, may occur at any time, and is not due to the fit of the lens or its design. The foreign body does not always cause pain (the patient may not even be aware of its presence), does not create visual disturbances, and may lodge in the superficial or middle epithelial layers.

Contact lenses may protect the cornea from such foreign bodies as welding sparks, grit, and debris. However, small, gritty particles such as mascara and dust can be carried beneath the lens by the tears and may become embedded in the cornea while contact lenses are worn. The nonperforating injuries they cause usually affect the epithelial layers exclusively, rarely penetrating Bowman's layer.

When fluorescein is used, an irregular film line in the area of injury may be noticed. The dye will penetrate the epithelium according to the extent of the corneal invasion. There is edema in the surrounding areas of the wound, and its edges are relucent. After the foreign body is removed, epithelial regeneration is rapid.

In penetrating wounds, all the corneal layers are traversed by the foreign body; in nonperforating wounds, the opening does not extend toward the anterior chamber and there are no healing problems. Corneal scarring and other problems may occur when Bowman's layer is penetrated.

Dixon[25] has stated that faint scratches in the epithelial surface made by foreign bodies that float into the eye and lodge beneath corneal lenses are common and can be considered normal.

A black-light fluorescein examination prior to biomicroscopy will expose a bright, deep, intense fluorescence where the foreign body is embedded in the epithelium. There is lighter, less intense fluorescein staining in the surrounding edematous areas. Colorless minute foreign bodies such as glass are difficult to observe. However, foreign bodies in the epithelium usually stain with fluorescein and are properly diagnosed with biomicroscopy, using sclerotic scatter and diffuse illumination. Direct illumination, narrow beam, is used to determine the depth of penetration. Retro-illumination and indirect illumination are used to examine the surrounding areas for epithelial edema. Specular reflection is used to examine the affected area for physical characteristics of the material. Contact lens wear should be discontinued until the foreign body is removed and healing has occurred.

CHANGES IN CORNEAL CURVATURE AND REFRACTIVE STATUS

The cornea can be considered a dynamic variable that reacts to physical pressures. Therefore, it is not surprising when changes in corneal curvature and refractive status are found immediately after contact lenses are removed; the quantitative changes are related to time.

After the patient becomes a contact lens wearer, it is good procedure to record corneal curvatures for each principal meridian and to refract the eye using static retinoscopy and a subjective examination during every patient visit. These values should be recorded as a permanent part of the patient's fitting history, and reference should be made to them as long as the patient remains a contact lens wearer.

Ophthalmometers are designed to measure curvatures from a convex corneal surface; biomicroscopes are used for objective examination of the cornea for physiological or anatomical changes. The functions of these instruments should not be confused. It is possible that the emphasis placed on ophthalmometer changes may be related to an assumption among contact lens practitioners that the contact lens fit is a good one when the flatter corneal meridian curvature changes are within plus or minus 0.50 diopters of the prewear values.

A contact lens may affect the cornea mechanically, often

through friction and swelling in the areas affected by lens movement. When there are nonuniform corneal bending (corneal deformation) and corneal thickness changes, there is corneal edema. Thus central keratometric changes make it appear as if only the central corneal areas are bending and the posterior contact lens surface is creating a forming effect on the corneal front surface. An increase in corneal thickness is either a major factor or a secondary result of the bending.

All this emphasizes the need for measuring the apparent corneal thickness prior to fitting contact lenses as well as during all followup and aftercare visits. After this information has been assembled for a representative number of contact lens wearers, perhaps it will be possible to correlate corneal curvature and refractive changes with corneal metabolic changes so that etiologic factors can be identified.

Frequently, the spectacles worn by the patient prior to the contact lens fitting are inadequate; and although new prewear spectacles had been prescribed they were never fitted. Therefore, it is important that at all clinical visits the patient's vision be measured and the findings recorded with the original as well as the immediate prewear spectacle prescription after contact lenses are removed. Additionally, the patient should be refracted with static retinoscopy and subjective, or manifest, examination techniques so the immediate spectacle prescription and visual acuity can be determined.

The results of static retinoscopy immediately after contact lens removal are unpredictable, inconsistent, and usually different from the pre–contact lens wear findings. In some instances, retinoscopy reveals dark, irregular, arcuate areas, often contained within what appears to be an impression of the contact lens on the cornea and resembling the retinoscopic scissors usually found in corneal dystrophy and keratoconus. Yet the ophthalmometer mires may be clear, there may be no significant corneal curvature changes, the patient may report no symptoms of discomfort, and the biomicroscope examination may show an absence of corneal interference.

A standard subjective examination is made, monocularly and binocularly, to learn if the patient's vision can be corrected to prewear levels. The new spectacle prescription is compared with the spectacle prescription worn by the patient on the first visit to the office for contact lens fitting and with the spectacle prescription determined when the patient was examined for contact lens wear.

It is generally assumed that the contact lens fit is good only when the patient's vision with the prewear conventional spectacles returns to prewear levels within 30 to 60 minutes after contact lens wear is discontinued. However, in many cases, when the patient's prewear spectacles cannot correct the vision to prewear levels immediately after contact lens removal and a new spectacle prescription must be used, this does not negate an otherwise good fit as long as prewear vision levels can be obtained with some form of spectacle prescription.

Visual acuity should be corrected to prewear levels with some form of conventional spectacle prescription that is determined immediately after contact lenses are removed. Although visual acuity may vary, the refractive state eventually stabilizes so that the patient is able to interchange contact lenses and conventional spectacles without a loss of visual acuity.

When vision cannot be corrected to prewear levels with some form of spectacle prescription immediately after contact lenses are removed, major corneal interference should be suspected. The interference is generally caused by a Grade 2 or Grade 3 corneal epithelial edema, with or without an increase in corneal astigmatism, that is greater than 1.00 diopter. This situation dictates a need for corneal rehabilitation.

Procedures designed for corneal rehabilitation prior to the availability of gas-permeable contact lenses inconvenienced patients from 2 to 3 weeks because contact lens wear had to be discontinued until the edema was reduced and the refractive state stabilized. An alternative procedure was to prescribe a reduced wearing schedule to satisfy corneal rehabilitation needs.

It is fortunate that gas-permeable contact lenses are available and can be prescribed for immediate refitting and corneal rehabilitation. Silicone elastomer contact lenses have been prescribed for this purpose when there were no marked corneal astigmatic increases; CAB and Polycon firm corneal lenses have been used in other situations. The ability of these materials to transmit oxygen and satisfy lacrimal interchange beneath the lens allows immediate refitting without inconvenience.

NOTES

1. J. K. Fitzgerald, *Oxygen Performance of Contact Lens Materials* (paper presented at Optifair West, Los Angeles, California, September 28, 1978).

2. J. B. Goldberg, "Gas Permeable Contact Lenses—How Good Are They?" *International Contact Lens Clinic* 6 (December 1979): 281–287.

3. R. C. Tripathi, "Applied Physiology and Anatomy: Tears, Cornea, Conjunctiva, and Ocular Adnexa," in *Contact Lens Practice,* ed. M. Ruben (New York: Macmillan, 1975), pp. 24–55.

4. M. A. Lemp and J. R. Hamill, Jr., "Factors Affecting Tear Film Breakup in Normal Eyes," *Archives of Ophthalmology* 89 (1973): 103–105.

5. S. Duke-Elder and A. G. Leigh, "Corneal Degenerations, Dystrophies, and Pigmentation," in *System of Ophthalmology,* vol. 8, ed. S. Duke-Elder (St. Louis: C. V. Mosby, 1965), pp. 957–976.

6. P. D. Bergenske, "Krukenberg's Spindle and Contact Lens–Induced Edema," *American Journal of Optometry and Physiological Optics* 57 (December 1980): 932–935.

7. J. B. Goldberg, "Ellipsoidal Corneal Lenses," *Optometric Weekly,* May 22, 1975, pp. 442–445; J. B. Goldberg, "Some Characteristics of Ellipsoidal Corneal Lenses," *Optometric Weekly,* November 13, 1975, pp. 1098–1099; J. B. Goldberg, "Eccentricity Values of Corneal Lenses," *Optometric Weekly,* April 1, 1976, pp. 340–342.

8. J. M. Dixon, "Ocular Changes Due to Contact Lenses," *American Journal of Ophthalmology* 58 (September 1964): 423–424.

9. R. B. Mandell, *Contact Lens Practice: Basic and Advanced* (Springfield, Ill.: Charles C. Thomas, 1965), p. 23.

10. J. H. Doggart, *Ocular Signs in Slit Lamp Microscopy* (St. Louis: C. V. Mosby, 1949).

11. Dixon, "Ocular Changes Due to Contact Lenses."

12. Doggart, *Ocular Signs in Slit Lamp Microscopy.*

13. M. L. Berliner, *Biomicroscopy of the Eye* (London: Hamish Hamilton Medical Books, 1949).

14. Ibid.

15. Ibid.

16. S. Duke-Elder and A. G. Leigh, "General Pathological Considerations," in Duke-Elder, *System of Ophthalmology,* vol. 8, pp. 671–675.

17. H. H. Boyd, "Two-Day Adaptation to Contact Lenses," in *Corneal and Scleral Contact Lenses,* ed. L. J. Girard (St. Louis: C. V. Mosby, 1964), pp. 366–371.

18. P. F. White and D. Miller, "Corneal Edema," *International Ophthalmology Clinics: Complications of Contact Lenses* 21 (Summer 1981): 3–12.

19. R. L. Farris, G. H. Takahashi, and A. Donn, "Corneal Oxygen Flux in Contact Lens Wearers," in Girard, *Corneal and Scleral Contact Lenses,* pp. 413–425.

20. L. N. Kline and T. J. DeLuca, "Corneal Staining," *International Ophthalmology Clinics: Complications of Contact Lenses* 21 (Summer 1981): 13–26.

21. J. M. Dixon and E. Lawaczeck, "Corneal Dimples and Bubbles under Corneal Contact Lenses," *American Journal of Ophthalmology* 54 (November 1962): 827–831.

22. F. Dickinson, "Some Corneal Changes Associated with Wearing Contact Lenses," *British Journal of Physiological Optics* 17 (1960): 161–170.

23. Dixon and Lawaczeck, "Corneal Dimples and Bubbles."

24. M. Schapero, "Tissue Changes Associated with Contact Lenses," *American Journal of Optometry* 43 (August 1966): 477–499.

25. Dixon, "Ocular Changes Due to Contact Lenses."

Chapter 7

Biomicroscopy in Determining Firm Corneal Lens Modification Procedures

An important advantage in using biomicroscopy in contact lens practice is that diagnostic information that can be used as a guideline for contact lens modification is obtained. Biomicroscopy can be used to assess a lens fit at any time, but it is impractical to modify a firm corneal lens fit when there has been under 4 hours of wearing time unless the fit is obviously improper.

When intermediate-zone bearing, peripheral bearing, and limbal impingement interfere with gaseous and lacrimal interchange, edematous areas of the central corneal epithelium and punctate lesions are formed. Similarly, corneal insult occurs when apical bearing interferes with lacrimal interchange in the central corneal area and restricts the removal of metabolic wastes. Therefore, lens modifications should be made to improve the tear pump and more evenly distribute bearing pressure. However, it is not always possible to determine in advance how the lens-cornea fit will be changed when corneal lenses are worn for all waking hours.

Contact lenses are classified by type, fitting philosophy of the practitioner, shape or design, structure, and physical chemistry (material). Lens type is determined by the size of the lens and the number of ocular curves; there are monocurve, bicurve, and multicurve lenses. The various types of lenses are made from a basic monocurve lens; the number of curves added is related to the corneal topography and the fitting philosophy.

Corneal lens shapes and designs may be the same—for example, toric or aspheric base curves or bifocal corneal lenses. Their structure will be either firm or slightly flexible, and their material will be either gas-permeable or non-gas-permeable.

SILICONE ORGANIC COPOLYMERS
The availability of hydrogel contact lenses changed the status of contact lens materials, causing an immediate reduction in the use of firm corneal lenses made of polymethylmethacrylate (PMMA).

The PMMA lenses have survived so far, although there has been a pronounced reduction in the number of new contact lens patients fitted with them. However, the survival of conventional PMMA material is now being seriously threatened by new materials that transmit oxygen. The physiochemical properties of these new materials resemble those of PMMA. The major difference is their Dk values (amounts of oxygen permeability).

Gas-permeable firm corneal lenses are usually slightly more comfortable than PMMA lenses initially and have a faster adaptation time. They eliminate such problems as photophobia, glare, surface drying, and afterwear refraction changes. They preclude the development of corneal edema when they satisfy the clinical criteria of a good lens-cornea fit. They also have certain disadvantages, however. They are more brittle than PMMA lenses and more easily scratched, have less dimensional stability, and flex more in response to digital pressures and handling, thereby reducing visual acuity. Also, identical materials vary in oxygen transmissibility, and some of the lenses may not be modifiable because of destruction of the wettability characteristic, which would preclude continuing comfortable wear.

The ideal fitting situation for gas-permeable corneal lenses is knowledge of the Dk value of the lens material, the power, the posterior lens surface specifications, the characteristics of tear flow under the lens, the cornea's demand for oxygen, and the lens thickness over its entire diameter.[1] We may be several years away from using such a modality in contact lens practice; however, the fitting of silicone elastomer contact lenses may be close to satisfying the prerequisites of a good physiological contact lens fit wihthout knowledge of how much oxygen a cornea demands.

It may be incorrect to assume that a Dk value is always a constant for contact lens materials. The value can vary between batches and along the rod (when the material is cast in rod form) so that a button cut from the bottom of a rod can have a slightly lower Dk value than one that is cut from the top of the rod.[2] Thus for gas-permeable corneal lenses the material might be suspect when it is necessary to reject a good physical fit because of corneal edema. Temperature changes also change the Dk value, which increases as temperatures rise.[3]

Should material wettability be included with oxygen transmissibility and lacrimal interchange as a property that is critical for successful corneal lens fitting? Edwards[4] states that the efficiency of tear circulation improves with better surface wetting, a situation that helps assure a good corneal physiological state when lens thickness reduces the amount of oxygen transmissibility. The Contact

Lens Manufacturing Association (USA) Standards Committee has standardized a method of measuring the wetting angles of corneal lens surfaces.[5] However, although the method of measurement is a constant, the wetting angle values can be changed by the manufacturing and polishing methods, the material's properties, the type of liquid used on the lens surface for the measurement, the age of the material when the measurement is made, and whether the measurement is made when the material is completely dry or after it has been allowed to soak.

For example, the Boston lens has a lower than usual wetting angle when the measurement is made after a representative soaking period. Tighe[6] quantified the wettability of the Boston lens not by the wetting agent but by the prewear soaking solution; he did not, however, describe the prewear soaking time involved. A presoak of the lenses in a solution buffered to a slightly alkaline pH appeared to improve wettability by as much as 20 percent. The wetting angle is 68° when the lenses are stored dry but measured with water. When Tighe's results are compared to the wetting angle found when the lenses are stored dry, they do not dictate a need to presoak the material. It may be impractical for contact lens manufacturers to send lenses to practitioners in a wet state. However, it may be practical for practitioners to soak the lenses prior to fitting them.

So far, the availability of several types of gas-permeable contact lens materials has either decreased or eliminated many corneal physiological fitting problems. Lens powers between plus and minus 3.00 diopters apparently do not dictate a need to seek an average thickness for effective oxygen transmissibility.[7] Although decreasing lens thickness for gas-permeable corneal lens materials will increase oxygen transmissibility, it will also increase lens flexing and dimensional instability when the lens is not supported structurally.

Firm corneal lenses are made in different center thicknesses, ocular surface shapes, and materials. Very thin PMMA corneal lenses flex on digital pressure. So do gas-permeable firm corneal lenses when their centers are too thin for the prescribed power.

Firm corneal lenses are usually fitted with corneal alignment regardless of the base curve shape—for example, spherical, aspheric, or toric. They are designed to be positioned either on the geometric center of the cornea or slightly above it. A low lens position is undesirable because the lens can become immobile and can induce corneal edema and subsequent lens rejection.

Polycon corneal lenses were originally fitted with apical bearing. This type of fit caused the lenses to be positioned above the geometric center of the cornea (a high lens position) and to move appreciably on blinking, as if they had literally been fastened to the upper lids. The early fitting method was later changed by making the lenses smaller, fitting them with corneal alignment, and allowing practitioners to custom design them.

A good lens-cornea fit and an edge-lift that satisfies lacrimal interchange needs are prerequisites for clinical success regardless of the amount of oxygen a material transmits. Although a corneal lens material can transmit oxygen in an amount that should satisfy the cornea's demand for oxygen when a lens is worn, corneal edema can develop when a poor lens-cornea fit is created by an immobile lens position, insufficient lens movement on blinking, and a too deep tear reservoir under the edge. Biomicroscopy is used to examine the contact lens fit for position, movement or displacement on blinking.

Gas-permeable corneal lens materials are similar to each other only in that they all transmit oxygen. The amount of oxygen transmissibility varies according to the polymeric formulation and center thickness of the lenses.[8] When compared with conventional and modified PMMA lenses, gas-permeable firm corneal lenses fit more securely (preferably with corneal alignment, perhaps with larger overall lens sizes). Also, their positions are hardly ever changed on blinking, although they are displaced slightly.[9]

PMMA corneal lenses have trade names that identify them according to their overall lens size and center thickness. Gas-permeable corneal lenses are instead identified by the commercial names of their materials. Their lens design variables are controlled according to FDA protocols. Consequently, the standard design of a gas-permeable corneal lens is established by the material manufacturer, which submits lens design variables to the FDA for approval. However, a practitioner can order a custom designed gas-permeable corneal lens.

Contact lens practitioners probably use the clinical procedures for fitting PMMA corneal lenses as guidelines for developing individual rationales for fitting gas-permeable corneal lenses. Some practitioners fit gas-permeable lenses according to the contour (alignment) fitting philosophy. The lenses are made from 0.2 mm to 0.5 mm larger than PMMA lenses as a way to control lens centration and displacement on blinking. However, the optic zone diameter is kept at 7.5 mm regardless of the base curve radius value. The diameter is made smaller when it is necessary to reduce or eliminate the degree of para-apical corneal bearing.

It is no longer judicious for practitioners to consider using large or small corneal lenses in general. Instead, clinical investigation is needed to determine the overall lens size that is best for the patient. This investigation is especially meaningful when fitting the currently available gas-permeable corneal lenses.

A corneal lens is fitted according to its relationship to the corneal diameter and the palpebral fissure. For example, the lens may be fitted within the corneal diameter (intracorneal diameter fit), and this fit can be either a between-the-lid fit (interpalpebral fissure fit) or an under-the-lid fit.

When the overall lens size is the basis for selecting design variables, without regard to clinical consideration of the patient's immediate needs, fitting problems that preclude comfort and clinical success may result. Therefore, practitioners should consider the interrelationships that exist between all the lens design variables and their relationship to the fitting philosophies. Although lens size and center thickness values have often been emphasized, more emphasis should be given to the ocular surface design of corneal lenses.

The size of a corneal lens is determined by the relationship between lens power, center thickness, and ocular surface shape. Spherical base curve corneal lenses can be made thinner than toric base curve lenses, for example. Very thin flexible PMMA corneal lenses have reduced or eliminated many clinical problems and have expanded the service life of the lenses. However, gas-permeable corneal lenses made with silicone have a tendency to flex when normal center thickness values are used. The result is an anachronism. Making contact lenses thinner is a way to increase oxygen transmissibility. A gas-permeable corneal lens that flexes on the eye may create many corneal physiological problems, however. Therefore, gas-permeable corneal lenses are made thicker than their PMMA counterparts.

Spherical base curve corneal lenses dominated the first 25 years of the modern contact lens era (1950–1975). In that period only a slight effort was made to fit toric base curve shapes, and few practitioners fitted aspheric base curves. Consequently, many poor lens-cornea relationships were created; also, when spherical base curves were used to fit large amounts of corneal astigmatism, many fitting failures occurred. A spherical base curve can be used effectively when the lens is made from PMMA materials and the corneal astigmatism does not exceed 2.50 diopters. It can also be used effectively when the lens is made from silicone organic copolymers or CAB materials if the corneal astigmatism does not exceed 1.75 diopters. Firm corneal lenses made from silicone organic copolymers are not as rigid as those made from PMMA materials and consequently flex more. Corneal lenses that flex appreciably when they are worn will adhere to the corneal surface in some degree, will leave an imprint or impression on the cornea, may be difficult to remove, and frequently will create significant edema (but without increasing the corneal astigmatism more than 1.25 diopters).

The overall corneal lens design and the relationship between the base curve shape (design) of the lens and the corneal topography are meaningful regardless of whether the material is gas-permeable. Permeability alone cannot be depended on to provide the entire oxygen supply to the cornea when the lenses are worn; the tear pumping mechanism will remove corneal metabolic wastes and furnish oxygen to the cornea. Selecting a gas-permeable firm corneal lens material is a way to eliminate marginal fitting problems; it is not a solution to major problems. Corneal lenses with low gas permeability may satisfy the cornea's oxygen needs when the lens-cornea fit is good and lacrimal exchange occurs.

SILCON HARD RESIN CORNEAL LENSES

Silcon hard resin corneal lenses are 100 percent silicone polymer. They are rigid, optically clear and stable, mechanically strong, and gas-permeable, transmitting nearly 50 percent of available oxygen in the atmosphere at sea level. The amount of oxygen they transmit is acceptable for cosmetic or aphakic extended wear. However, the lenses may flex when worn, and they cannot be modified without their wettability being destroyed.

Practitioners can use the same biomicroscope procedures to fit silcon hard resin corneal lenses that are used to observe and evaluate PMMA or silicone acrylate hard corneal lenses. Silcon hard resin lenses are effective for up to 1.50 to 1.75 diopters of corneal astigmatism. Because their centers are thinner than those of silicone elastomer lenses, they will flex and induce unwanted residual astigmatism when the corneal astigmatism is progressively greater than 1.50 diopters. They will flex more quickly and to a greater degree when they are fitted with pronounced apical clearance so that peripheral clearance at the edge is reduced and the lens adheres to the corneal surface in the periphery. This situation will create an impression of the lens on the corneal surface that can be observed with biomicroscopy when the lens is removed (see Figures 7-1 and 7-2). Therefore, silcon hard resin corneal lenses must be fitted with good peripheral corneal clearance.

The results of a poor lens-cornea fit can be seen when the lens is removed by examining the cornea with diffuse illumination, low and high magnification, and the blue filter, if the tears are stained with fluorescein. A stagnant apical tear pool beneath a gas-permeable lens can cause corneal edema and epithelial linear formations in the apical area; the severity is related to time (see Figure 7-3).

Figure 7-1. Diffuse illumination, low magnification, showing an aspheric multifocal Silcon corneal lens fit with apical clearance. The lens is secure on the cornea and centered well over the pupil.

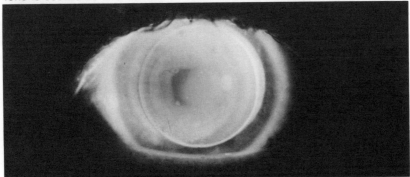

Diffuse illumination, low magnification, is used for general observation of the lens-cornea fit. Direct illumination, medium and then narrow band, low magnification, is then used to assess the depth of the central dye pool. Direct illumination, low magnification, medium and narrow beam, is used to focus on the dye patterns at the periphery under the peripheral curve. If the characteristics of clearance and bearing areas are to be observed and assessed, the

Figure 7-2. Diffuse illumination, high magnification, showing an impression left by the Silcon lens on the cornea and epithelial edema and staining over the pupil. Arcuate peripheral corneal staining is seen at 7 to 11 o'clock.

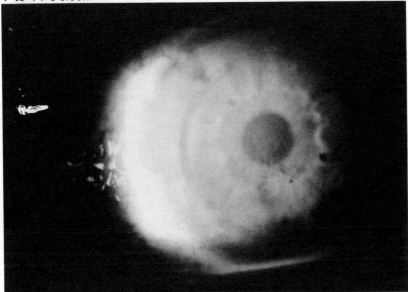

Figure 7–3. Direct illumination, medium beam, low magnification, showing epithelial edematous linear formations in the apical area.

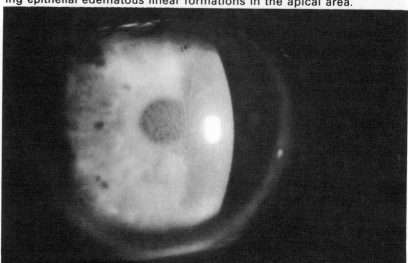

microscope is moved from a temporal to a nasal area and the angle of the incident light is changed by moving the stage of the instrument. The focus is adjusted as needed.

When corneal problems occur, the lens should be redesigned for a better lens-cornea fit. A flatter spherical base curve can generally be used. However, when the corneal astigmatism is progressively greater than 1.50 diopters, a toric or aspheric base curve should be used.

Mechanically induced peripheral corneal edema and abrasions may occur shortly after the patient begins all-day wearing. These problems occur when the cornea wets poorly because the tear breakup time is too rapid. A combination of corneal drying in the peripheral areas and lens movement causes peripheral corneal edematous changes, epithelial denudation, and staining. The affected areas frequently coalesce to form a corneal abrasion. It is possible to reduce the severity and degree of peripheral corneal staining by blending spherical peripheral curves or by changing to an aspheric curve.

Diffuse illumination, low and high magnification, is used to observe the wetting characteristics of the anterior surface of the corneal lens when it is worn. The surfaces are examined for lipid or protein deposits that may accumulate on them. These deposits inhibit wetting and cause discomfort. Poor surface wetting is also caused by Meibomian secretions on the lens surfaces and by chemical reactions of the lens materials and tears.

Although removing the surface deposits with a surfactant cleaner will improve surface wetting, there is no dependable way to improve wetting when the cornea tends to become dry. Corneal dryness can be the result of an aqueous or mucin deficiency in the tears, and gas-permeable lens materials often do not correct the problem. Neither hydrogel nor silicone organic copolymer materials seem to reduce or eliminate the clinical problems caused by corneal dryness. However, some practitioners have found that CAB contact lens materials reduce the degree of discomfort and corneal interference.

Grosvenor[10] lists the following criteria for contact lens design:

1. The base curve should be essentially parallel to the central portion of the cornea, thereby preventing the lens from exerting pressure on the sensitive corneal apex. Also, the lens should have little effect on the tarsal conjunctiva.
2. The peripheral portion of the ocular lens surface should be flattened sufficiently to allow adequate exchange of tears and gases beneath the lens. It should fit loosely enough that blinking will move it up and thus further aid in this exchange.
3. The optical zone of the lens should be large enough to keep the lens well centered in front of the patient's pupil but not too large to keep it from lagging during a blink.

Grosvenor[11] also states:

Normal physiological functions including sensitivity, transparency, water transfer and transfer of oxygen and carbon dioxide must be taken into consideration in the designing of a contact lens. Even though such optical and physical factors as visual acuity and comfort, corneal topography and adequate centration are of great importance, the final test of a contact lens depends upon the extent to which it is compatible with corneal physiology.

Contact lenses must satisfy the functional needs of patients by ensuring (1) maintenance of uninterrupted lacrimal interchange (venting), (2) absence of limbal impingement and scleral encroachment for all quadrants, and (3) apical clearance, whether alignment is minimal or pronounced.

Patients' clinical needs, which are not quite as important as their functional needs, are satisfied by the following:

1. The anatomic features and the metabolism of the cornea and adnexa must not be disturbed.
2. The patient must be not only comfortable but also visually efficient when wearing the contact lenses.

3. Visual acuity must be restorable to normal limits with conventional spectacles after lens removal.

4. The surface and edges of the lens must be scratch-free and highly polished so that movement caused by lid pressure will not disturb the integrity of the epithelial surface or irritate the perilimbal capillaries.

5. The optical element of the corneal lens should be oriented over the pupil, without peripheral curve encroachment, so that the patient will not experience monocular diplopia, flaring, or ghost images.

6. The lens should not move beneath the lower lid.

7. There should be minimum vertical displacement and change of position during blinking.

CONTACT LENS DESIGN VARIABLES

The effectiveness of a contact lens fit is determined by the individual dimensions of each design component as well as by the interrelationships of the various design components or variables. The lens should be comfortable and visually efficient, it should be oriented over the pupil, and it should not interfere with corneal metabolism or corneal transparency. The components of contact lens design are (1) base curve and optic zone diameter, (2) intermediate and peripheral curve radii and their widths, (3) lens diameter, (4) lens center thickness, (5) edge contour and thickness, and (6) power.

Several clinical procedures can be used to determine the initial variables of the contact lens design: nontrial lens fitting, trial lens fitting, and fitting from inventory sets. When a nontrial lens fitting method is used, the ophthalmometer measurements and spectacle prescription are sent to a laboratory. Measurements of the corneal diameter, pupil diameter, vertical palpebral fissure dimensions, and position of the lower lid as it relates to the inferior limbus may also be sent. The laboratory will design a contact lens on the basis of this information and will send it to the practitioner, who must then assess its clinical effectiveness by evaluating the patient's adaptation to it. This method provides a corneal lens design that will correct visual acuity and maintain a relatively good position; however, there is no assurance that it will result in the best lens design.

A more exact (and preferred) method is trial lens fitting, which uses the ophthalmometer measurements and the spectacle prescription as reference points in observing the clinical performance of a series of diagnostic lenses. This method can be expanded to allow the practitioner to fit the patient immediately when there is a representative contact lens inventory of base curves and lens powers.

An inventory fitting set of corneal lenses is convenient. It is also important for fitting aspheric multifocal corneal lenses, whose clinical success is achieved only when the lens fit satisfies centration and movement criteria.

Regardless of the fitting method or philosophy used, practitioners need to know how to modify contact lens design variables. In making the appropriate modifications when corneal insult occurs because of incorrect design, practitioners can be guided by biomicroscope findings and by knowledge of the functions of lens design components. The necessary corrective procedures may be simple modifications or may involve entirely new lens designs.

If the same lens is used, the modification may consist of one or more of the following: reduction in lens size, reduction in the optic zone diameter (which is the equivalent of widening the peripheral curves), flattening of the peripheral curves, power changes of plus or minus 0.50 diopter or less, and the addition of venting fenestrations. A new lens is required for the following modifications: change in base curve, change in power more than plus or minus 0.5 diopter, increase in overall lens diameter, increase in optic zone diameter, increase in curvature of the peripheral curves to a steeper or shorter radius, and change in center thickness.

Base Curve and Optic Zone Diameter

The *base curve* is critical since it is related to prescription needs and apical clearance. Daily and Daily[12] consider the term *diameter,* when applied to contact lenses, to be synonymous with either the width of a curve or the greatest distance across the lens. It is not twice the radius of curvature.

The *optic zone diameter,* then, is the chord diameter of the base curve. It is the physical difference between the overall lens diameter (lens size) and the width of the peripheral curves, and it forms the major portion of the overall lens diameter.[13] It is almost always made larger than the central corneal zone (optic cap) and pupil.[14] Thus it is a critical variable for apical clearance when it is altered and the base curve is either retained or changed. Table 7–1 shows the effect on the lens fit of changes in design components.

Peripheral Curves

The peripheral curve is a nonoptical curve that has a longer radius than the base curve and is fabricated on the ocular surface so that it replaces the base curve in the peripheral areas. The radius of the peripheral curve allows the lens to stand farther away from the cornea at its edge and thus to furnish an adequate reservoir of tears. The peripheral curve is made flatter than the base curve (0.5 mm minimum difference) so that it extends from the lens periph-

Table 7-1 Lens Fit after Modification of Design Components

Base Curve	Optic Zone	Apical Clearance	Lens Fit
Steeper	Constant	Increased	Tighter
Steeper	Larger	Increased	Tighter
Steeper	Smaller	Not changed or slightly reduced	Not changed
Flatter	Constant	Reduced	Looser
Flatter	Larger	Not changed or slightly increased	Not changed
Flatter	Smaller	Reduced	Looser

ery toward the center to form the optic zone diameter, and its width is one-half the difference between the overall lens size and the optic zone diameter.

Lens types are defined as follows: a *bicurve lens* has one peripheral curve and a base curve, a *tricurve lens* has two peripheral curves and a base curve, a *quadricurve lens* has three peripheral curves and a base curve, and a *pentacurve lens* has four peripheral curves and a base curve. Although lens types are easily distinguished by this classification, there is no standardization of the nomenclature for peripheral curves. Manufacturers and contact lens practitioners use different terms in identification and classification. For example, the nonoptical curve in the peripheral areas of a bicurve lens may be known as a *bevel curve* or as a *secondary curve*. Similarly, when more than one nonoptical peripheral curve is used, the curves may be classified according to their position on the ocular surface.

For a contact lens ocular surface, a flatter radius always replaces a steeper radius. Thus for a base curve of 7.8 mm (43.25 diopters), a peripheral curve of 9.3 mm (1.5 mm or approximately 7.50 diopters flatter than the base curve) will replace the base curve until the manufacturing process ends. A distinctive junction between the curves allows easy measurement of the curve widths. When a third curve is used, for example, 8.5 mm (0.7 mm flatter than the base curve), it will replace more of the area on the ocular surface occupied by the base curve and will obscure the junction formerly present between the base curve (7.8 mm) and the 9.3 mm peripheral curve, but it will not form an appreciably visible junction between its width and the 9.3 mm curve because the physical difference is slight. Thus, when the junctions between peripheral curves are obscured, the lens is a *blended lens;* the blending is classified according to the quality (light, medium, or heavy, for example). Although this is not a particularly good classification, it has become an established frame of reference for practitioners and manufacturers.

Some use the indicated procedure to fabricate peripheral curves on an ocular surface of a contact lens; others use a different technique. For a base curve of a 7.8 mm radius, peripheral curves of 8.5 mm and 9.3 mm may be required. When the 8.5 mm curve is fabricated first and the 9.3 mm curve is fabricated later, there will be visible junctions between all ocular surface curves. When additional curves having intermediate radii are used to obscure the junctions formed between curves, what classification should be given to the curves and the lens type? This problem is for those experienced in working with design standards; it is beyond the scope of this text.

The arbitrary selection of the number of peripheral curves is related to the lens design (bicurve, tricurve, and so on) and to the overall lens size. The term *secondary curve* refers to a curve that is just peripheral to the optical zone of a contact lens and is usually made 0.6 to 1.2 mm longer than the base curve. The most peripheral curve is classified as the bevel, or peripheral, curve; it is much narrower and flatter than the secondary curve, and has a radius of 11.5 or 12.5 mm.

The peripheral (or secondary) curve radius and number should be based on fitting needs. A peripheral curve made 1.5 mm flatter than the base curve has been found best for standardization in almost all the fitting philosophies. Occasionally, a peripheral curve made 1 mm flatter than the base curve has been used to reduce lens movement and to make the lens fit more secure. It has not been necessary to use a peripheral curve more than 1.5 mm flatter than the base curve to make the lens fit less securely; instead, when it has been necessary to improve venting to reduce apical clearance or to loosen the lens fit, the optic zone diameter has been made smaller or the peripheral curve width wider by using a peripheral curve radius 1.5 mm flatter than the base curve.

Peripheral curve widths are decreased when their radii are more than 1.5 mm (approximately 7.50 diopters) longer than the base curve. Their widths are increased when their radii are less than 1.5 mm flatter than the base curve in order to allow the lens to stand closer to the cornea.

When the peripheral curve radius is a constant for all base curves, the difference is a variable. When the difference between the peripheral curve radius and the base curve is a constant, the peripheral curve radius is a variable. For example, with a standard 12.25 mm peripheral curve used for all base curve radii, when the base curve is 7.5 mm, the difference is 4.75 mm; and when the

Table 7–2 Effect of Alterations in Peripheral Curve Radius and Peripheral Curve Width

Peripheral Curve Radius	Peripheral Curve Width	Lens Fit
Flatter	Constant	Looser
Flatter	Increased	Looser
Flatter	Decreased	Not changed
Steeper	Constant	Tighter
Steeper	Increased	Not changed
Constant	Increased	Looser
Constant	Decreased	Tighter

base curve is 8 mm, the difference is 4.25 mm. Conversely, with the use of a 1.5 mm difference between peripheral curve and base curve radii, when the base curve is 7.5 mm, the peripheral curve is 9 mm; and, when the base curve is 8 mm, the peripheral curve is 9.5 mm. Alterations in peripheral curve radius and width produce changes in the lens-cornea relationship, as Table 7–2 shows.

Since different methods are used in manufacturing peripheral curves, there are often differences in the fit of corneal lenses made by different laboratories—although the peripheral curve tools used may theoretically have the same radius. Therefore, practitioners should consistently use the trial lenses made by one laboratory.

One of several methods can be used to generate and polish a peripheral curve radius. The radius can be (1) lathe-cut and polished on the basic lens blank before the uncut lens is manufactured; (2) cut on the basic lens blank before the uncut lens is manufactured and then polished on the uncut, or unfinished, form; (3) generated on the uncut, or unfinished, lens with either diamond- or carborundum-covered radius tools and then polished; (4) polished completely on the uncut, or unfinished, lens form without prior lathe cutting or grinding.

Because the center thickness of the lens blank is not appreciably reduced when a peripheral curve radius is generated and polished on the basic lens blank, the lens is not subjected to the molecular stress and strain that occur when the radius is generated on an uncut, or unfinished, corneal lens in this particular manufacturing process. Lathe cutting and pitch polishing of the peripheral curve radius may be a more exacting, more expensive, and optically superior manufacturing method, but it may also result in fitting delays because the lens must be returned to the laboratory for modifications unless the practitioner is equipped to make laps with pitch- or wax-covered tools in the office.

Peripheral curves can be polished with radius tools covered

with pitch, polishing wax, or such softer materials as adhesive tape (waterproof and nonwaterproof), velveteen, felt pads, foam rubber, or silk. When a peripheral curve tool is covered with pitch or polishing wax, the thickness of the material does not change the radius of the peripheral curve. The exact peripheral curve radius can be generated on a tool either by lathe cutting after the pitch or wax is cooled or by forming when the pitch or wax is slightly warm.

When a peripheral curve tool is covered with a material other than pitch or polishing wax, the thickness of the material covering the tool makes the peripheral curve radius flatter by the amount of its thickness. The thickness of the material should be measured, and the peripheral curve radius should be made steeper in the amount of the thickness of the material so that the radius will have the proper clinical value after it is polished. The tool is then said to be *compensated.* Thus, for a peripheral curve radius of 9 mm, a radius tool of 8.7 mm is used when the thickness of the covering material is 0.3 mm. However, the material will become thinner with wear; therefore, unless the pad is changed after each use of the tool, the results will not remain constant.

Although spherical peripheral curves are generally used to finish corneal lenses, an aspheric peripheral curve can also be used for this purpose. Aspheric peripheral curves become progressively flatter toward the lens edge throughout their width and are identified by their degree of edge-lift: normal, less than normal, and flatter than normal. Changing the aspheric peripheral curve, or bevel, values will not change the central fitting characteristics of the lens but can be used to improve lacrimal interchange under it or to control a poor edge-lift situation. An inherent advantage of the aspheric peripheral curve is its assured reproducibility; it is made with one tool.

Aspheric peripheral edge finishing is restricted to a curve width of 0.6 mm because of the aspheric design. Thus an aspheric peripheral curve can be used in addition to one or more spherical peripheral curves to create an aspheric bevel, a corneal lens finishing feature that reduces lens awareness and enhances comfort.

Lens Diameter

The sum of the widths of the optic zone diameter and the peripheral curve widths is the lens diameter. The fit of the lens is changed when its overall diameter, or lens size, is changed. Alterations in lens size can be made with or without changes in either the optic zone diameter or base curve or with any combination of changes. Such changes affect the lens position and fit, as shown in Tables 7–3 and 7–4.

Table 7-3 Effects of Modifications of the Lens Size and the Optic Zone Diameter

Lens Size	Optic Zone	Effect
Smaller	Constant	Makes lens fit more secure. Displaces optic zone slightly higher so that its edge moves nearer to the inferior pupil margins. Reduces the amount of lens stock that encroaches on the superior sclera and impinges on the superior limbus. May reduce lens movement.
Smaller	Smaller	Makes lens fit less secure. Decreases apical clearance. Reduces para-apical bearing and obstruction to lacrimal interchange in the intermediate zones. May increase lens movement.
Smaller	Larger	Makes lens fit more secure centrally. Increases apical clearance. Improves lens centering over pupil and may eliminate lens impingement on superior limbus and lens encroachment on superior sclera. Prevents peripheral areas of lens from encroaching on pupil areas. (Removes flaring, ghost effects, and monocular diplopia.) May eliminate or reduce vertical displacement.
Larger	Constant	Makes lens fit more secure. Eliminates lagging of lens. Improves meridional orientation.
Larger	Smaller	Makes lens fit more secure, although lens position may be slightly higher. Reduces apical clearance. Reduces amount of para-apical bearing. Eliminates lagging of lens.
Larger	Larger	Makes lens fit more secure. Increases apical clearance. Prevents peripheral areas from encroaching on pupil areas. (Removes flaring, ghost effects, and monocular diplopia.) Eliminates lagging of lens. Improves meridional orientation.

Table 7–4 Effects of Modifications of the Lens Size and the Base Curve

Lens Size	Base Curve	Effect
Constant	Steeper	Makes lens fit more secure. Increases apical clearance. Reduces vertical displacement. Improves lens centering over pupil.
Constant	Flatter	Makes lens fit less secure centrally. Reduces apical clearance. Reduces amount of intermediate zone bearing and removes obstruction to lacrimal interchange in para-apical corneal areas. (Improves venting.)
Larger	Constant	Makes lens fit more secure. Improves geometric centering of lens on cornea. Reduces lens movement.
Larger	Steeper	Makes lens fit more secure. Increases apical clearance. Improves lens centering over pupil. Reduces lens movement.
Larger	Flatter	Makes lens fit less secure centrally but more secure generally. Reduces apical clearance. Improves lens centering over cornea. Reduces amount of intermediate zone bearing and removes obstruction to lacrimal interchange in para-apical corneal areas. (Improves venting.)
Smaller	Constant	Reduces amount of lens stock that encroaches on the superior sclera and impinges on the superior limbus. Displaces optic zone slightly higher so that its edge moves closer to the inferior pupil margins. May reduce lens movement.
Smaller	Steeper	Makes lens fit more secure. Increases apical clearance. May increase para-apical zone bearing. Reduces amount of lens stock that encroaches on the superior sclera and impinges on the superior limbus. Improves centering of lens over pupil.
Smaller	Flatter	Makes lens less secure peripherally and centrally. Reduces apical clearance and intermediate zone bearing. Improves intermediate zone venting. May cause lens to lose geometric centering on cornea.

Because several methods are used in fitting contact lenses, no attempt has been made here to numerically quantify the changes in design variables involved in the various modification procedures. Thus the arbitrary descriptions provided are intended only to suggest the direction of change; they do not represent a precise indication of the results in the individual situation.

Edge Contour and Thickness

An important aspect of fitting corneal lenses is the quantitative value of the edge thickness and contour. When the contour fitting philosophy is employed, lens edges are made between 0.18 and 0.22 mm thick. The edges are rounded, although they are not necessarily tapered.

Corneal lenses whose overall sizes are less than 9 mm and that are fitted within the corneal diameter (and sometimes between the lids) are more comfortable when their edges are tapered and thin. The contour should begin to taper at a point 0.15 mm from the lens edge; the thickness is between 0.12 and 0.1 mm at this point. The tapering gradually reduces the thickness to approximately 0.03 mm at the extreme edge, which must be rounded and highly polished for comfort.

The quality of the edge finishing can be assessed by microscopic inspection. The contour of the edge and its thickness can be measured with a shadow profile comparator that has a millimeter measuring scale.

Although the edge shape just described has proved the most successful in some practices, each practitioner has a concept of what constitutes a good edge shape. What is considered optimum by one practitioner will be totally rejected by another. This seems paradoxical when one considers how much emphasis is usually placed on obtaining a good edge shape. Two biomicroscope methods can be used to inspect lens edges: direct magnification and projection magnification.

Direct Magnification Procedure

1. Using low or high magnification, open the biomicroscope diaphragm to its maximum width.
2. Hold the lens either between the fingers or in a small-diameter suction cup (or a holder that will not obscure the lens edges).
3. Look through the microscope, moving the lens closer and farther away, up and down, until it is in focus.
4. View the lens edge that is visible, and observe the contour of the edge as the lens is tilted and slowly moved closer and

farther away. Rotating the lens, repeat this procedure until the entire edge has been inspected.

5. Inspect the lens edge for lathe marks (poor polishing), scratches, indentations or elevations, and appropriate edge contour design.

Projection Magnification Procedure

1. Reduce the room illumination.
2. Using low or high magnification, open the biomicroscope diaphragm to its maximum width.
3. Hold the lens either between the fingers or in a small-diameter suction cup (or a holder that will not obscure the lens edges).
4. Move the lens closer to and farther from the microscope until a shadow of the edge is in focus on either an adjacent wall surface or a small white paper mounted on a wall near the microscope.
5. Slowly rotate the lens and observe the edge contour.

This method can be successful as described; however, it is enhanced when used with the projection shadow-profile magnifier.

Comment is in order for practitioners who assess the quality of a finished corneal lens edge by rotating the lens edge around their tongues or by placing the lens on their eyes to determine if the edge is finished properly. The first procedure is unsanitary and cannot provide the objective results obtained with instruments designed for the purpose. The results of the second procedure are influenced by individual corneal sensibilities. The technical and scientific advances in contact lens practice have made unhygienic and primitive procedures unnecessary.

LENS FIT PROBLEMS AND CORRECTIONS

Whatever fitting philosophy is involved, the lens-cornea relationship will be affected if the lens fit is too secure centrally, too loose centrally, too secure peripherally, too loose peripherally, or any two of these clinical problems. When a contact lens contours the cornea only in certain areas to support the lens position and pulls radially away from the corneal surfaces in other areas, the fit provides proper venting. A corneal lens fit is unsatisfactory if it exactly matches the corneal contour, because it interferes with lacrimal flow, allows retention of metabolic wastes, and reduces the oxygen supply to the cornea.

Because corneal topography cannot be measured exactly with current instrumentation, corneal reaction to contact lens wear is assessed after lenses are removed by keratometric examination, biomicroscope examination, and refraction. Now that pachometers are available, practitioners can also keep a chronological record of corneal thickness changes induced by corneal lens wear. However, in the absence of pachometry, refractive changes found when doing an after-refraction can also be used to estimate the degree of corneal edema. When corneal swelling is 6 percent or more, there will be visible corneal edematous changes. Therefore, slight myopia increases and hyperopia decreases found during an after-refraction can be used to assess the degree of corneal physiological changes when no changes are found with biomicroscopy.

Lens Fit That Is Too Secure Centrally (Spherical Base Curve)
A lens fit that is too secure centrally is produced by an apical clearance lens that has one or more of the following characteristics (see also Figure 7–4):

1. The base curve is too steep.
2. The optic zone diameter is too large.
3. There is excessive bearing in the intermediate corneal areas.
4. The peripheral curve is too steep.

Figure 7–4. Direct illumination, broad beam, high magnification, showing apical clearance pool and para-apical corneal bearing. The para-apical bearing can cause corneal edema and corneal curvature and refraction changes although the material transmits oxygen. The width of the peripheral curve is narrow at 8 o'clock, where the lens is beginning to adhere to the corneal surface.

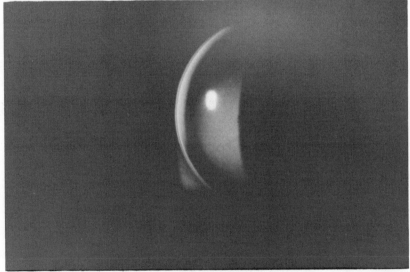

This fitting situation creates poor lacrimal interchange under the lens. It will cause corneal physiological changes regardless of whether the material is gas-permeable. Although a contact lens material may transmit oxygen, this property will not satisfy all the criteria for a good fit when the lens-cornea relationship restricts lacrimal flow and corneal metabolic wastes are retained under the lens.

Clinical Findings

The lens appears firmly fixed in position over the pupil. Only minimum vertical displacement upward or downward occurs during blinking, and the lens usually retains its position of geometric orientation over the cornea. Characteristic findings of black-light fluorescein examination are apical pooling, bearing areas in the para-apical corneal zones, and a continuous band of fluorescein tinted tears around the peripheral lens areas. After the lenses have been worn 4 hours or more, bubble retention can be observed beneath the central lens areas. When the bubbles coalesce, corneal abrasion may result. The patient usually experiences burning, stinging, and other forms of visual distress. After the lenses are removed, it is often difficult for the patient to achieve prewear levels of visual acuity with conventional spectacles. Interference with visual acuity experienced after contact lens removal has been called *spectacle blur*. A symptom of metabolic interference, it may persist for several minutes or several hours and sometimes can be eliminated with a different spectacle prescription.

There are several ways to refit a patient whose corneas need rehabilitation. Two methods were used when PMMA was the only material available:

1. Contact lens wear was discontinued until the corneal curvatures and refractive state stabilized; then, on the basis of new ophthalmometric and refractive data, the patient was refitted for new lenses.
2. The wearing time was reduced by 1 to 2 hours daily until lens wear could be discontinued completely; then, on the basis of new ophthalmometric and refractive findings, the patient was refitted.

Now that gas-permeable materials are available for contact lenses, it may not be necessary to use either the complete or partial withdrawal methods for corneal rehabilitation. Silicone elastomer contact lenses can be used for immediate refitting when the corneal astigmatism is not much greater than 2 diopters, and gas-permeable firm corneal lenses can be used regardless of the amount of corneal astigmatism. Both types of materials can provide a satisfactory sight vehicle while the cornea recovers from a severe hypoxic state.

Although gas-permeable corneal lens materials also induce cor- neal physiological changes when they fit on the cornea with strong, focalized bearing and restrict lacrimal flow, the degree of corneal edema is usually not as severe as it is when PMMA lenses are used. Also, the flexing characteristic of silicone organic copolymer materials may reduce the strength of the corneal bearing forces so that the degree of spectacle blur is less pronounced than it is with PMMA materials, the refractive and corneal astigmatic in- creases induced by contact lens wear are not as severe as with PMMA materials, and the myopic increases and hyperopic decreases rarely exceed 0.75 diopter. Practitioners who do an after-refraction at each office visit during the fitting procedure will quickly modify the contact lens design variables and will thereby eliminate the possibility of ever needing to rehabilitate a cornea. This technique is especially effective when the amount of corneal swelling is not great enough to cause visible biomicroscope changes.

The factors of apical clearance and a zone of para-apical bearing may create interference with lacrimal interchange beneath the lens and induce metabolic changes. The stagnant bubble formations be- neath the lens usually indent the epithelium. Biomicroscopy is used to detect apical bearing, lacrimal interchange deficiencies, and ep- ithelial dimpling and edema.

Procedure for Evaluating an Apical Clearance Fit

1. Use sclerotic scatter and diffuse illumination to examine the bubble formations in the central areas beneath the lens for size, position, and movement and to study their surrounding areas.
2. Change to direct illumination, medium beam. While the micro- scope is focused on the tear layer (this is simplified when the tears are tinted with 2 percent sodium fluorescein), traverse the tear layer from the temporal to the nasal areas and observe clearance and bearing areas. Focus the microscope on the areas of bubble formation; alternately use indirect illumination and retro-illumination to examine for epithelial edematous areas.
3. Remove the lens and examine the eye for corneal edema, using sclerotic scatter and direct illumination. Also examine the ar- eas of epithelial staining with an optic section, and determine their depth. There may be small, localized, irregularly shaped areas of epithelial edema. The edematous areas will appear

grayish-white and cloudy and will be slightly obscured when there is no staining.

Characteristically, the apical clearance design does not produce bubble retention, stagnant central lacrimal pooling, and epithelial dimpling. A small lens may fit firmly in position, geometrically centered over the cornea, and its narrow width of para-apical bearing may not interfere with lacrimal interchange. However, in some cases, the lens fit may be improper but appear to be normal when examined with fluorescein and black light, and biomicroscope examination may not expose edematous areas or interruption of the epithelial surfaces. After the lens is removed, however, dark, irregular arcuate areas contained within what appears to be an impression of the contact lens on the cornea can be observed with static retinoscopy. Ophthalmometer measurements may be as much as 0.75 diopter steeper for the flatter primary corneal meridian, and visual acuity equal to prewear levels may be unobtainable. It would be correct to assume in this case that the lens fit is too secure and has induced corneal changes.

Modification Procedures

Apical clearance and the width of the para-apical bearing areas must be reduced to eliminate interference with lacrimal interchange. It may be judicious to make these changes in small amounts so the effect of each change can be observed. If further modifications are required, they can be continued until the problem is corrected. When the optic zone diameter is decreased, apical clearance and the width of para-apical bearing areas are reduced.

To reduce the optic zone diameter, the existing secondary curve radius, a flatter one (from 0.3 to 0.5 mm flatter), or an aspheric peripheral curve to improve venting is used. When the optic zone diameter is to be reduced so that the modification does not create a major change of the lens position, a radius of curvature that is slightly steeper than the existing peripheral curve and slightly flatter than the base curve can be employed. The peripheral curve tool used for this procedure is covered with a soft material (velveteen or silk) to blend the transition angles between curve junctions. This modification will reduce the optic zone diameter and automatically increase the width of the peripheral curves when the lens size remains constant.

The optic zone diameter can be reduced by 0.3 mm when the lens size is less than 9 mm and by 0.5 mm when it is more than 9 mm; the reduction will work especially well if the lens has a contour fit. It is questionable whether the fitting problem will be eliminated if the optic zone diameter is reduced in amounts less than these values.

Another method of making the lens fit less securely is to reduce the overall lens size by 0.2 mm to 0.4 mm. Also, a series of flatter peripheral curves or an aspheric peripheral curve can be used to increase edge-lift and facilitate lacrimal interchange. In the modification of the peripheral lens edges, the procedure of using a flat radius first and then progressively steeper radii will automatically reduce the transition angles between curves and obscure their definition (blending). The peripheral lens areas will then have several flat curves with small widths and minimum edge standoff and thus will aid in venting. This procedure can also be used with an aspheric peripheral curve.

To produce a parabolalike edge contour, a series of radii of 17 mm, 15 mm, and 12 mm are used (in this order), all of them being 0.1 mm wide. The successful fabrication of a parabolalike edge design depends on the presence of sufficient lens stock. A lens may have insufficient edge thickness to allow this modification to be made successfully, since the use of flatter curves at the peripheral areas may remove plastic and reduce the overall lens size. Therefore, this type of modification may necessitate the fabrication of a new lens with a center thickness great enough to permit the overall lens size to be retained.

When it appears that a further reduction of the optic zone diameter will cause the inferior lens edge to encroach on the pupil, it will be necessary to make a new lens with a base curve that is flatter by at least 0.5 diopter (approximately 0.1 mm). This procedure will reduce apical clearance and provide a larger optic zone diameter. When the base curve is made flatter, the lens power must be compensated in the amount and direction of the change.

Lens Fit That Is Too Loose Centrally (Spherical Base Curve)
A lens fit that is too loose centrally is produced by a lens that has one or more of the following characteristics:

1. The base curve is too flat.
2. The optic zone diameter is too small.
3. The peripheral curves are too flat or too wide.
4. The lens size is too small.
5. The center thickness is too thick for the power.

Clinical Findings
The lens may be positioned on or slightly below the inferior limbus. The lens edges may stand away from the peripheral corneal areas

Figure 7-5. Direct illumination, broad beam, high magnification, showing bubble formations under the peripheral lens area of a corneal lens displaced downward on blinking.

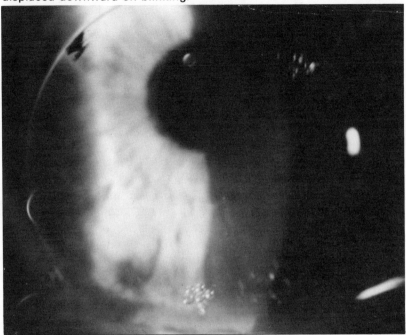

and thus may produce bubble formations and stagnation beneath the central areas (see Figure 7-5). When part of the lens is covered by the lower lid, there is interference with lacrimal interchange and gaseous exchange. A base curve that is too flat or an optic zone diameter that is too small, or both, may produce apical bearing. Although a lens is fitted according to the alignment, apical bearing may develop when the flatter corneal curve becomes steeper in the early months of wear or when the lens base curve flattens.

Apical bearing causes a looser lens fit. Excessive lens movement induced by the blink may produce small punctate abrasions (stippling) or irregular epithelial abrasions without form or pattern. When an edematous epithelial area adjoins an area of stippling or abrasion, severe corneal abrasions and ulceration may result.

Black light and fluorescein show marked peripheral clearance and deep fluorescence; the apical areas are dark. Occasionally, irregular epithelial staining is observed. The patient may be more aware of the lens, although no pain or other distress is experienced. However, there may be a photophobia, burning, and stinging. The lens may move off the cornea or out of the eye. Vision with conventional spectacles after contact lens wear is usually less than before contact lens wear.

Procedure for Evaluating an Apical Bearing Fit

1. For biomicroscope examination while the lens is worn, tint the tear layer with sodium fluorescein and use direct illumination, medium beam, low and high magnification, to traverse the cornea. Focus the microscope on the tinted tear layer and observe apical bearing areas, which appear as dark areas without fluorescence. Use sclerotic scatter with low magnification and diffuse illumination, indirect illumination, and retro-illumination with low and high magnification to observe the movement of lacrimal debris and the formation and retention of small bubbles in the apical areas.

2. After the lens is removed, use diffuse illumination, indirect illumination, and retro-illumination with low and high magnification to examine the limbal vessels for engorgement and to see any extension of the limbal vessels to the corneal peripheral areas. Examine the perilimbal vessels with diffuse illumination, low and high magnification. Have the patient change fixation approximately 10° to 15° temporally. Then reduce the width of the beam and change the angle of incident light to approximately 45° to 60° temporally. Use indirect illumination and retro-illumination, low and high magnification, to examine the limbal vessels in the nasal portions of the cornea. Then, reversing the procedure, examine the limbal vessels in the temporal corneal portions. Repeat this procedure using the red-free filter.

3. Use diffuse illumination and indirect illumination with low and high magnification to detect areas of corneal epithelial erosion, which have any one or more of the following characteristics: (a) a series of small punctate lesions within the apical bearing area; (b) epithelial edema in the immediately adjacent areas, which appear as grayish-white irregular lines; (c) denudation of the corneal epithelium (stained areas). Wearing the lens without modification may induce further epithelial changes, such as deep abrasions, edema, and corneal ulceration.

Modification Procedures

1. For lenses made with a spherical base curve, restore apical clearance with a new lens that is designed to increase the sagittal depth. The most immediate way to eliminate apical bearing is to make the base curve 0.50 diopter (usually 0.1

mm) steeper with prescription compensation and to retain the other lens design variables.

2. When the lens is positioned either on or below the inferior limbus or below the corneal center, make the new lens size larger (by either 0.3 mm or 0.5 mm) in combination with the procedures just described, or keep the lens base curve a constant. Reducing the center thickness will also reduce lens movement and improve centration.

3. When the center thickness is too great for the power, the lens is moved across the cornea by the blink. A new lens, made thinner by 0.02 mm to 0.03 mm, may produce a more secure lens fit. The center thickness value of the thinner lens must be compatible with the overall lens size, the power, and the width and radius of the peripheral curve. Since an alteration in center thickness may also change the characteristics of the edge thickness and design, it may be advisable to use a lenticular construction when it is necessary to reduce the center thicknesses for certain powers so that the thickness and design of the edge can be retained—for example, for plus power lenses.

As a special construction feature, the new lens can be made with a pronounced minus lenticular carrier that will allow the upper lid to grasp the lens and hold it in a more central position. This lens can be used for either plus or minus powers.

It is preferable to fit a firm corneal lens so that it is centered over the cornea or positioned slightly above its center, it fits on the corneal surface with the best possible uniform bearing, and it is moved only slightly on blinking so that it does not mechanically disturb the corneal epithelial surface. These basic principles apply to all firm corneal lens materials, regardless of their oxygen transmissibility.

Lens Fit That Is Too Secure Peripherally (Spherical Base Curve)

A lens fit that is too secure peripherally shows areas of peripheral bearing and is usually high riding; part of the lens covers the cornea, and part impinges on the superior limbus or encroaches on the superior sclera. The cause is any one or more of the following:

1. The overall lens size is too large.
2. The base curve is too flat.
3. The peripheral curves are too wide or too flat, with the result that excessive edge standaway causes the lens to be displaced upward by the blink.

Corneal lens materials made with silicone will flex on the eye. A combination of a pronounced apical clearance fit and the flexing characteristics of the material may cause the lens to fit securely on the peripheral corneal areas. Severe peripheral corneal bearing pressures will create an impression of the lens on the corneal surface that can be observed with biomicroscopy when the lens is removed.

Clinical Findings
The lens is fixed in position high on the cornea. There is insufficient peripheral clearance in the areas where the lens impinges on the superior limbus. This situation frequently causes the limbal vessels to fill and to proliferate onto the peripheral corneal areas. Occasionally, there is also conjunctival injection.

The high lens position is characteristic of an on K fit for corneal astigmatism of 2.00 diopters or more (spherical base curve lens), especially for a lens of high minus power. When the lens position is high, the optic zone diameter often encroaches on the lower pupil areas and the patient may report visual distress with monocular diplopia.

A high lens position is also characteristic of a Polycon corneal lens that is fitted with a base curve made flatter than the flatter corneal curve, an overall lens size of 9.5 mm, and an optic zone diameter of 8.4 mm. When the lens is made in minus powers, the upper lid will grasp it and raise it. The lens may also move with the upper lid on blinking. This type of fit may not be offensive to practitioners who prefer to have the upper lid move the lens across the corneal surface on blinking. However, the lens may also retain an immobile high corneal position when it flexes and the degree of flexure offers resistance to the blinking forces.

Procedure for Evaluating a High Lens Position

1. Stain the tears with fluorescein and use the previously described system of filters to observe the lens fit with the biomicroscope.
2. Use diffuse illumination or direct illumination, broad and medium beam, low and high magnification, to examine the fit for corneal bearing and clearance areas.
3. Use sclerotic scatter, low magnification, to observe the lens position.
4. Raise the upper lid slowly and observe the position of the superior lens edge. Usually it will rest on the superior scleral areas, and there will be an absence of fluorescein under the lens in these areas. In fact, there will be dye stained tears under the

peripheral lens edge where the lens covers the cornea; the tears generally disappear in the superior limbal areas where the lens bridges the superior corneal-limbal junction.

The patient may be aware of the lens during blinking when the lens edge is thick and round, square and sharp, or thin and poorly polished or when it stands away from the eye appreciably and forms an oblique angle at the edge apex (ski-nose edge shape). Tear stagnation may cause photophobia, burning, and stinging.

A lens positioned at too high a level will induce epithelial edema, stippling, dimpling, and superficial vascular changes in the superior limbal areas. Bimicroscope examination with sclerotic scatter, low magnification, will expose stagnant bubble formations beneath the lens. With this technique:

1. Use diffuse illumination, low and high magnification, to examine the bubble formations and the lacrimal pooling in the superior corneal quadrants:
2. Examine the bubble spacing and observe changes in the position of the bubbles when the upper lid is retracted and the patient looks down.
3. Study the appearance of the superior limbal vessels to detect differences from the findings of the biomicroscope examination made before fitting.
4. After instilling fluorescein with the lens in place, use direct illumination, medium beam, low and high magnification, and focus the microscope on the tear layer. Traverse the cornea and examine for apical clearance and bearing areas. Examine for limbal vessel proliferation as well as for general perilimbal vascular changes by means of indirect illumination, retro-illumination, diffuse illumination, and direct illumination, medium beam, low and high magnification.
5. After the lens is removed, examine the areas of epithelial dimpling with direct illumination, medium beam; and with an optic section, narrow beam, low and high magnification, determine their depth.
6. Use indirect illumination and retro-illumination, low and high magnification, to examine corneal edematous areas.

Modification Procedures

The modification often employed first is reduction in overall lens size, with all other design components retained. The peripheral curve width is thus automatically reduced. Although the reduction in size may correct the lens impingement on the superior sclera, it may also raise the lens relative to the pupil. As part of the same modification, the lens edges can be made thinner, thus removing the tendency of the upper lid to grip the lens and move it upward. (In plus lenticular constructions this problem is minimal.)

Although this modification may be successful, the individual clinical condition should be the guide in making any change. As a general rule, a high lens position is the result of improper base curve selection; it occurs when a spherical base curve is fitted on K to correct with-the-rule corneal astigmatism in excess of 1.50 diopters. The lens is in alignment with the flatter horizontal corneal meridian, its edges stand away from the steeper vertical meridian, and the blink moves the lens upward. This fitting problem can be corrected by using a steeper base curve (retaining the optic zone diameter or making it larger) and a smaller lens size or by replacing the spherical base curve with one that is either toric or aspheric; the lens will fit within the corneal diameter and, usually, within the palpebral fissure.

The spherical base curve is made from 0.50 to 1.00 diopter steeper, according to clinical findings. However, whenever possible, trial lenses should be used to determine the quantitative change. When the corneal astigmatism is greater than 2.50 diopters, toric base curves should be considered.

To facilitate lens centering, it may be helpful to make a new lens that has a larger optic zone diameter (between 0.3 and 0.5 mm), since apical clearance increases when the base curve dimension is retained and the optic zone diameter is increased. Sometimes the combination of a steeper base curve, a larger optic zone diameter, a smaller overall lens size, and a thinner center thickness may be necessary to center the lens over the cornea.

A prism ballast design with increased center thickness can be used to lower the lens. The prism is between 1 and 1.5 prism diopters. The base curve is made steeper, and the optic zone diameter is either retained or made larger, causing it to be displaced 0.5 mm above center toward the apex of the prism to center the optical element of the lens over the cornea. An unequal peripheral curve width is thus formed.

It might also be judicious to change from a firm corneal lens to a silicone elastomer or hydrogel contact lens. A silicone elastomer lens has greater structural strength and is slightly more rigid than a hydrogel lens. Therefore, a change from a firm corneal lens to a silicone elastomer lens will satisfy vision needs when the corneal astigmatism does not exceed 2.00 diopters. Of course, the corneal astigmatism will have to be less than 1.25 diopters for refitting with a hydrogel contact lens that will satisfy vision requirements.

The existing lens should be modified according to these suggestions to improve centration and eliminate lens encroachment on the superior scleral areas. Changing to a smaller, thinner corneal lens, preferably of gas-permeable contact lens material and with either a spherical, aspheric, or toric base curve (the latter can be prescribed when the corneal astigmatism is greater than 1.50 diopters) is another way to change from a secure, high-position lens fit to one that satisfies corneal centration and lacrimal interchange criteria.

Lens Fit That Is Too Loose Peripherally (Spherical Base Curve)
A fit that is too loose peripherally is produced by a decentered lens that has one or more of the following characteristics:

1. The base curve is too flat.
2. The optic zone diameter is too small.
3. The lens size is too small.
4. The peripheral curve is too flat.

The displacement of lenses may be due to corneal asymmetry, particularly decentration of the corneal apex and nonuniform corneal flattening. Although Polycon corneal lenses fit with apical bearing are deliberately designed to be loose in the periphery so that they can be moved by the lids on blinking, this section will deal only with firm corneal lenses whose fit is unintentionally too loose peripherally.

Clinical Findings
The lens does not center well. The displacement may be nasal or temporal, high or low. The peripheral areas often encroach on the pupil and induce visual disturbance. Often, the lens moves during blinking. Excessive lens movement may cause superficial epithelial disturbances such as punctates, stippling, and irregular linear staining. Occasionally, discomfort and visual distress result when mucous and lipid deposits form on the lens surfaces. Conjunctival injection may develop after relatively short periods of contact lens wear. The perilimbal vessels may become engorged and may proliferate into the peripheral corneal areas.

Lens movement may cause photophobia, lid irritation, and lid edema. The patient may report a need to squint to keep the lens from moving off the cornea or out of the eye.

Biomicroscopy will reveal the epithelial disturbances resulting from this type of poor fit, showing lacrimal interchange to be unaffected. Bubbles that migrate beneath the lens are quickly dispersed.

However, peripheral air pockets beneath the lens occasionally fill with a large bubble or several small bubbles; the latter may remain when the peripheral curve is too flat.

With the lens in place, sclerotic scatter and diffuse illumination are used to observe metabolic interference and deposits on the lens. Mucous particles may have various shapes and formations. Their movement pattern can be seen clearly after fluorescein staining. If the lens surface is coated with these particles, changes in surface wetting characteristics will be observed.

The metabolic disturbances that occur have various characteristics. Areas of epithelial denudation appear as irregular grayish-white sections on the corneal epithelial surface. They vary in depth and are usually present where apical bearing and excessive lens movement have affected the cornea. These areas will stain with flourescein. Punctates and stippling caused by lens movement can be found over various corneal areas. Conjunctival injection and irritation of the lid margins resulting from lens movement and poorly designed edges are examined with diffuse illumination (low and high magnification). With direct illumination, narrow beam, low and high magnification, an optic section is used to evaluate the relationship between the corneal periphery and the peripheral curves.

After the lens is removed, all abraded corneal areas are examined with direct illumination, narrow beam, low and high magnification, to determine the depth of the abrasion. Indirect illumination and retro-illumination, low and high magnification, are used to examine epithelial edematous areas (which appear grayish-white when they are part of the erosion complex and stain with sodium fluorescein) and changes in the perilimbal vessels.

Modification Procedures

A new lens is usually required to provide centration over the pupil and cornea. It must have a larger overall size or larger optic zone diameter, with or without steeper base curves, a minimum center thickness, and thin, tapered edges. The modification of lens dimensions may consist of one or more of the following changes: (1) overall lens size larger by 0.3 to 0.5 mm, (2) base curve steeper by 0.50 diopter or more and with prescription compensation, (3) optic zone diameter larger by 0.3 or 0.5 mm, and (4) values of the peripheral curve and its width adjusted as indicated by biomicroscope evaluation.

The judicious use of trial lenses or lenses from an inventory fitting set will quickly establish whether the direction of change must be made for a steeper base curve, a larger lens size, or some combination of the two as a way to increase sagittal depth and eliminate the clinical problems. Although gas-permeable firm corneal lenses can be steeper and larger than PMMA lenses,[15] it is preferable to fit gas-permeable corneal lenses using the same guidelines used for PMMA corneal lenses. An alignment dye pattern and uniform corneal bearing areas are sought. Although they can be created with spherical base curves when the corneal astigmatism is progressively less than 2.50 diopters, sometimes the need is more easily satisfied with an aspheric base curve made from gas-permeable or PMMA materials.

The similarity between corneal topography and the aspheric corneal lens base curve shape makes it possible to use a larger lens size than that used for a spherical base curve. As for the aspheric base curve radius, it is always made slightly steeper than the flatter corneal meridian, a clinical situation that lends itself to an edge-to-edge alignment fit.

Corneal Edema Induced by Gas-Permeable Corneal Lenses

Gas-permeable corneal lens materials are both an asset and a liability. Their clinical value is determined by how they are fitted and managed. Practitioners cannot rely exclusively on the oxygen transmitted by a contact lens material to control the incidence and degree of corneal edema. They must first create a good lens-cornea relationship. A contact lens will satisfy the dictates of a good lens-cornea relationship when it is fitted with a uniform pressure gradient on the cornea, there is minimal movement and lens displacement on blinking, and lacrimal interchange beneath the lens removes corneal metabolic wastes. Corneal edema induced by gas-permeable contact lenses can be of either mechanical or physiological origin.

Although lens movement for all lens types is critical for a good fit, the amount of movement on blinking is directly related to such aspects of the lens-cornea fit as alignment, apical bearing, and apical clearance. There is a greater amount of lens displacement on blinking when there is apical bearing; there is less displacement when the fit is changed to increase apical clearance and attempt an alignment fit or, for silicone elastomer contact lenses, to create a slight apical clearance.

Mechanically induced corneal edema can be caused by a flat base curve, excessive lens movement across the corneal plane, and pronounced edge lift (see Figure 7–6). Constant mechanical irritation of a corneal area may prevent the recovery of the epithelial cell, causing the area to become abraded and edematous. This situation can also be induced at a limbal area by a silicone elastomer contact lens with poorly fabricated edges. A combination of lens

Figure 7–6. Direct illumination, broad beam, high magnification, showing mechanically induced peripheral epithelial denudation caused by excessive lens movement. The edge-lift is pronounced, and dye stained tears protrude beyond the lens edge.

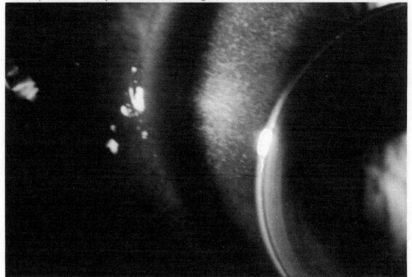

movement and poor edge fabrication may mechanically denude the corneal epithelium in a specific area, usually at the limbus, causing scattered corneal epithelial punctate staining in the central and peripheral corneal areas when there is poor lacrimal interchange under the lens. The spots of corneal edema in the peripheral area may coalesce to form a corneal abrasion.

Lens movement and corneal drying in the peripheral areas may create peripheral corneal edematous changes, epithelial denudation, and staining (see Figure 7–7). Epithelial denudation is observed with biomicroscopy, using diffuse illumination and direct illumination, medium and narrow beam, low and high magnification, in white light and with the blue filter and the yellow photographic filter when the tears are stained with fluorescein.

Physiologically induced corneal edema may be caused by a silicone hard resin corneal lens or a firm corneal lens made of silicone organic copolymer materials that flexes on the eye, causing the peripheral lens areas to adhere to the corneal surface and to leave an impression of the lens on the eye. Generally, the problem is caused by a steep base curve or a lens that is too thin to support the lens position and prevent it from changing when it is fitted for corneal astigmatism progressively greater than 1.50 diopters.

Pronounced and constant apical clearance may induce corneal edema and epithelial edematous linear formations over the pupil-

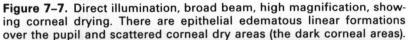

Figure 7-7. Direct illumination, broad beam, high magnification, showing corneal drying. There are epithelial edematous linear formations over the pupil and scattered corneal dry areas (the dark corneal areas).

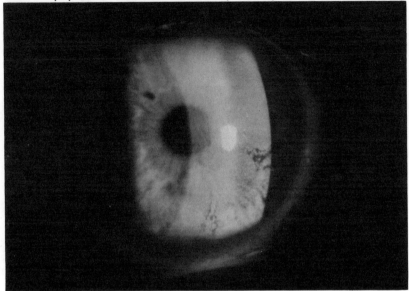

lary area. For pronounced apical clearance and strong, focalized para-apical corneal bearing forces, blinking may change the lens position slightly, but it does not necessarily move the apical clearance pool away from the pupillary area.

Tomlinson and Shoup[16] investigated the effect on corneal edema of variations in the base curve relationship of gas-permeable firm corneal lenses. Their objective was to learn the contribution made by the tear pump mechanism to the oxygen supplied with the contact lens and the degree to which oxygen transmission through the material was sufficient for the cornea's needs. Making the base curve of a hard corneal lens steeper increased corneal edema. However, the amount it was made steeper and its relationship to increasing corneal edema was one-half less for Polycon than for PMMA lenses.

A gas-permeable hard corneal lens can be fitted steeper than one that does not transmit oxygen—without creating corneal edema. However, the amount that it can be fitted steeper is a variable that is determined by the oxygen transmitted by the material. Regardless of the amount of oxygen a material can transmit, practitioners should fit gas-permeable contact lenses so that there is alignment in the corneal apical zone and minimal para-apical corneal bearing pressure.

The ability of a contact lens material to transmit oxygen and the availability of the tear pump to eliminate corneal metabolic debris form a critical relationship. The mathematical relationship that exists between the base curve of a corneal lens and the flatter corneal curvature can be considered a good one when the contact lens wear satisfies all clinical criteria for maintaining corneal transparency. Thus the base curve can be made steeper or flatter than the flatter corneal meridian. This is demonstrated with silicone hard resin corneal lenses. Fitting such a lens with pronounced apical clearance will preclude success when it physically interferes with the tear pump mechanism.

Lens flexing will cause central corneal epithelial edema and edematous linear formations when it interferes with lacrimal interchange and traps tears under the apical area. When the flexing is severe in the periphery, a circular stained area that resembles a corneal lens can be observed on the corneal surface when the lens is removed. This situation has occurred with silicone hard resin corneal lenses that are fitted with base curves that are too steep.

Biomicroscope techniques that can be used to examine the cornea for edema induced by gas-permeable contact lenses are diffuse illumination, direct illumination, medium and narrow beam, indirect and retro-illumination, low and high magnification, white light, and the blue filter and yellow photographic filter when the tears are stained with fluorescein. The biomicroscope procedures used to examine the cornea for edema are the same regardless of the contact lens material.

Although gas-permeable contact lenses may reduce the incidence and degree of corneal edema appearing with conventional PMMA lenses, they must also satisfy the criteria of a good fit: the absence of corneal edema, either no increases or only slight increases in corneal and refractive astigmatism (no more than 0.50 diopter for each), and refractive stability when the lenses are removed after a representative wearing period.

NOTES

1. J. Stone, "Designing Hard Lenses in the 1980's," *Journal of the British Contact Lens Association* 4 (April 1981): 130–137.

2. D. P. Auerbach, "Boston Lens," *Journal of the British Contact Lens Association* 4 (April 1981): 138–141.

3. K. H. Edwards, "Experience with XL20 (Calgary) and XL30 (Alberta)," *Journal of the British Contact Lens Association* 4 (April 1981): 142–144.

4. Ibid.

5. Contact Lens Manufacturing Association (USA) Standards Committee, *Standard Methods of Determining Wetting Angle (Chicago: Contact Lens Manufacturing Association, 1981).*

6. Reported in Auerbach, "Boston Lens."

7. I. Fatt, "A Comparative Study of Oxygen Transmissibility," *Contact Lens Forum* 6 (September 1981): 29–31.

8. J. B. Goldberg, "Gas Permeable Contact Lenses—How Good Are They?" *International Contact Lens Clinic* 6 (December 1979): 281–287.

9. M. E. Lees, "Polycon-CAB: A Clinical Comparison, *Ophthalmic Optician* 18 (1978): 816–819.

10. T. P. Grosvenor, "Physiological Factors in Contact Lens Wearing," *Optometric Weekly,* March 31, 1966, pp. 13–19.

11. Ibid.

12. L. Daily, Jr., and R. K. Daily, "Modification of Corneal Contact Lenses," *International Ophthalmology Clinics: Volume 1* (1961).

13. W. R. Baldwin and C. R. Schick, *Corneal Contact Lenses: Fitting Procedures* (Philadelphia: Chilton Book, 1962).

14. N. Bier, *Contact Lens Routine and Practice* (London: Butterworths Scientific Publications, 1957).

15. A. Tomlinson and A. C. Shoup, "The Effect of Fit of a Gas-Permeable Hard Contact Lens on Corneal Physiological Response," *Journal of the British Contact Lens Association* 4 (March 1981): 121–126.

16. Ibid.

Chapter 8

Biomicroscopy for Silicone Elastomer Contact Lenses

Silicone elastomer contact lenses are different from other contact lenses. They are not gel lenses. But their surface is hydrophilic. They are flexible, dry when off the eye, and wet when worn. They transmit large amounts of oxygen. They are more stable than hydrogel contact lenses and can be prescribed for corneal astigmatism up to 2 diopters.[1]

Silicone elastomer contact lenses are inert chemically and physiologically. They are extremely hydrophobic and must be treated so that their surfaces will become wet when they are worn. They are made of a synthetic material containing only silicone polymers, not natural rubber. Their water absorption is less than that of PMMA lenses. Their base curve and optics can be measured in air, using conventional hard corneal lens instrumentation. They transmit oxygen and carbon dioxide but not liquids. Consequently, they allow the cornea to retain its glycogen content within 4 percent of normal.

Silicone elastomer contact lenses can be damaged; however, they rarely tear, and they are difficult to scratch. They will not lose their elastic properties; hence their base curve will not warp with wear. Conventional small-molecule fluorescein can be used with black light or the blue filter in the slit lamp to assess and evaluate their fit.

Chemical and thermal methods can be used in cleaning and storing these lenses. It is not necessary to use thermal disinfection procedures (bacteria will not penetrate the material), but an enzyme cleaner or a surfactant cleaner that removes lipid and protein deposits may be useful at times. The lenses can be rinsed with tap water, and conventional hard corneal lens solutions can be used for wetting and storing them. However, none of the solutions should contain chlorbutanol, which will bind to the lens surfaces.

Perhaps the most important property of silicone elastomer contact lenses is their oxygen permeability. They have a Dk value of 340×10^{-11} at 21° C. This value means that they are thickness-independent for oxygen transmissibility. Furthermore, they will rarely induce neovascular changes, even with extended wear.

LENS COMFORT

A disadvantage that they share with hydrogel materials is that a decrease in visual acuity and comfort can occur when protein and lipid deposits develop on the surfaces, but the deposits can be removed with surface reactants. Perhaps a major disadvantage is their degree of initial comfort, which may resemble that of conventional hard corneal lenses, or, in some instances, be even less comfortable. Conventional hard lens wetting solutions do reduce the degree of initial awareness and discomfort, however. They furnish a lower surface wetting angle than do saline solutions.

Edge design and finishing characteristics also influence comfort and awareness.[2] Silicone elastomer contact lenses are molded with conventional male and female dies. High temperatures, pressures, and curing cycles are needed for vulcanization. The lens edges are ground mechanically and polished smooth by a patented process. Comfort is often a function of the effectiveness of the polishing at two places on the lens; the junction between the anterior central curve and the anterior peripheral curve on the front surface of the lens and the junction between the base curve and the peripheral curve on the ocular surface.

The degree of comfort further depends on the hydrophilic characteristics of the surfaces. Two processes can be used to change the surfaces from hydrophobic to hydrophilic. The objective is to reduce the surface wetting angle. The processes can be either electrochemical or chemical. The resultant wetting angle is comparable to that of other contact lens materials, about 50°.

Silicone elastomer contact lenses can be prescribed for corneal astigmatism up to 2.00 diopters, almost twice the range of hydrogel contact lenses. This feature allows them to be used in place of toric soft contact lenses in such situations. Of course, when prescribed as a sight vehicle for astigmatism, their oxygen permeability also allows them to be worn for extended wear. They can also be used to eliminate certain poor clinical situations caused by hydrophilic lens wear, among them vascular changes, conjunctival injection, hypersensitive reactions caused by soft lens solutions, persistent red eye, swollen lids, giant papillary conjunctivitis, and peripheral corneal vascularization.

Clinical Advantages

They have one important advantage over high-water-content hydrogel contact lenses prescribed for aphakic extended wear. Because they do not contain water, there can be none of the evaporation and resultant dehydration that exists for hydrogel lenses. Furthermore, their dry state allows them to retain their dimensional stability. Consequently, the incidence of corneal neovascularization and giant papillary conjunctivitis is rare. Because the material is thickness-independent for oxygen transmissivity, it could become the number 1 material for cosmetic extended wear for low plus powers. Although much has been written about silicone elastomer contact lenses for general use, their characteristics also allow them to be used effectively for such specific needs as instant refitting of myopic patients, who have advanced corneal edema induced by hard corneal lens wear but who are without major or pronounced increases in corneal astigmatism.

DYE PATTERNS

The dye patterns are used to observe the fit and clinical effectiveness of silicone elastomer contact lenses. An optimum fit should satisfy the following criteria: (1) lens centered or positioned slightly above center, (2) 1 mm lens movement on blinking, (3) continuous fluorescein tear film from edge to edge, (4) minimal apical clearance, (5) minimal intermediate (para-apical) bearing, (6) moderate edge-lift, and (7) stable overrefraction.

Diagnostic or inventory lenses must be used in fitting silicone elastomer contact lenses. The lens base curve is fitted from 0.4 mm flatter than the flatter corneal meridian to on K, on the basis of clinical observation of the trial lens fit. The lens power used is identical to the spherical spectacle power. The lens diameter is smaller than the corneal diameter.

Conventional black-light fluorescein diagnostic procedures can be used to assess and evaluate the fit. The observation can be made macroscopically or with a biomicroscope. However, the practitioner must wait for the initial tearing to subside before observing the fitting characteristics. This time period may be as long as 10 or 15 minutes.

Biomicroscopy Procedures for Silicone Elastomer Lenses (Figures 8–1 to 8–8)

1. Use sclerotic scatter, low magnification, to observe the lens position and movement on blinking. The lens should either be centered on the cornea or positioned slightly above center. Generally, it seeks a position that is slightly above center and displaced temporally, literally a slightly oblique up-and-out position.

Figure 8–1. Diffuse illumination, 16x, low magnification, showing the silicone elastomer contact lens almost centered over the cornea. This is a good geometric corneal position. The peripheral clearance is well defined, suggesting that the lens should be displaced slightly on blinking. The apical clearance and para-apical corneal bearing are typical of the way this lens fits on the eye. Although the lens is slightly displaced laterally when fixation is in the primary position, the relationship between the pupillary area and the central optical zone of the lens implies that there will be no visual distress created by the lens when it is displaced on blinking.

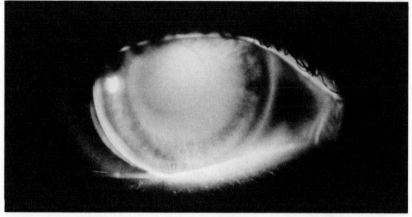

2. Slowly increase the width of the incident light beam, and observe the fit using diffuse illumination, low magnification. The lens should move on blinking, but the amount of movement should be minimal, not exceeding 2 mm.
3. Place one or two drops of fluorescein on the superior scleral area while the patient looks down. Place the blue filter in the slit lamp and, if it is available, place a yellow #2 photographic lens filter in front of the lens housing the microscope system. The lens-cornea fit can now be assessed and evaluated.
4. Position the slit lamp from 15° to 30° away from the examiner, and slowly change the angle of incident light as needed to obtain a full view of the lens on the cornea. Use diffuse illumination, low magnification, to observe the lens position, lens movement, and surface wetting characteristics.
5. Reduce the width of the incident light beam to form direct illumination, medium beam. Move the lens from one edge to the other while observing the characteristics of the dye patterns for clearance and bearing, noting their positions.

A silicone elastomer contact lens will fit well when it has good peripheral clearance and when the lens movement allows lacrimal

Figure 8-2. Direct illumination, broad beam, high magnification, showing lacrimal debris accumulations under a silicone elastomer contact lens. The base curve is too flat. Excessive lens movement has trapped lacrimal fluid in the apical area under the lens, and this fluid will cause corneal edema in the pupillary area.

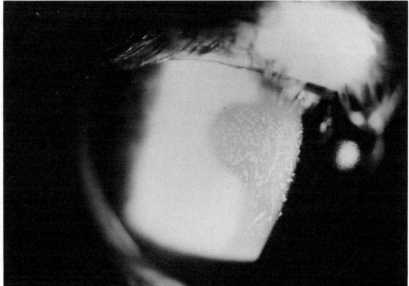

interchange beneath the lens to eliminate corneal metabolic wastes. Peripheral clearance is important. There should be a wide band of fluorescein beneath the lens circumference, but the lens edges should neither stand away from the ocular surface nor extend above the edge of the lower eyelid.

Although the flatter corneal curvature is used as a basis for selecting the base curve and although the base curve radii of the lenses have an appropriate relationship to it, the final selection of the base curve is determined by the appearance of the peripheral fit. It is because of this appearance that silicone elastomer contact lenses can be from 0.2 mm flatter than K to as much as 0.3 mm steeper than K. Final judgment for the base curve radius is made on the basis of observation of the dye patterns, preferably with a biomicroscope.

There may be a narrow annulus of corneal bearing between the peripheral curve area and the apical area. There should be a small amount of apical clearance, which may or may not change in volume on blinking. The lens should move on blinking, but the amount of movement should be minimal. Excessive lens movement may denude the corneal epithelial surface and induce a mechanical

Figure 8–3. Diffuse illumination, low magnification, showing a silicone elastomer lens that has been worn without removal for 4 weeks. There is good peripheral clearance and reduced apical clearance. There are two circular surface deposits; one is seen at 9 o'clock off the pupillary area, and the other is slightly obscured in indirect illumination at 3 o'clock. Removing the lens, cleaning it, and replacing it on the eye will restore a typical fluorescein fitting pattern. Lens wear can be resumed and extended wear continued when further biomicroscope examination of the eye with the lens removed confirms the absence of corneal edema.

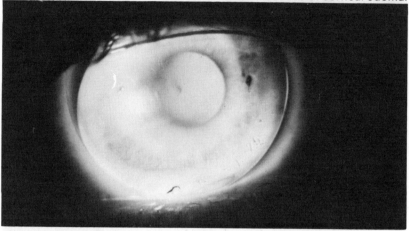

Figure 8–4. Diffuse illumination, low magnification, showing a type of surface deposit that forms on silicone elastomer contact lenses—a film that has various shapes and sizes. Deposits such as these can be examined further with direct illumination, broad, medium, and narrow beams, low and high magnification. The lens should be removed, cleaned, and replaced with a new one if cleaning does not restore a good optical surface and visual acuity.

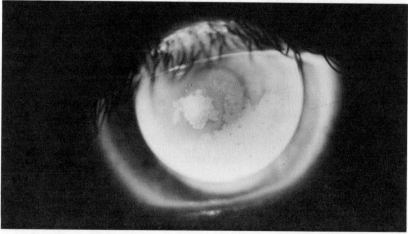

Figure 8–5. Direct illumination, medium beam, low magnification, showing a series of circular deposits that have formed on the surface of a silicone elastomer contact lens. There is also a larger circular deposit at 5 o'clock in the para-apical corneal area.

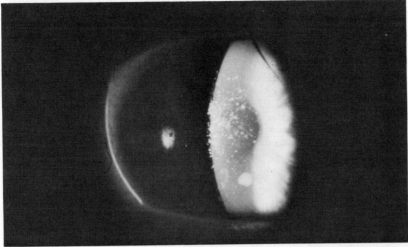

Figure 8–6. Direct illumination, medium beam, high magnification, showing the accumulation of surface deposits on the front surface of a silicone elastomer contact lens. There is also some specular reflection from the deposits. The larger single deposit is seen in retro-illumination, as are some of the deposits included in the accumulation.

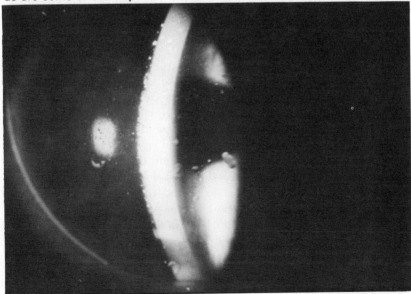

Figure 8–7. Poor surface wetting of a silicone elastomer contact lens and scattered corneal punctate staining. The poor wetting is seen as scattered dark areas in direct illumination, broad beam, low magnification.

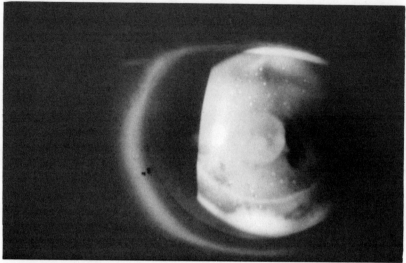

corneal abrasion at the limbal area. The corneal epithelium will stain, and in the peripheral area there will be scattered punctate stains that can coalesce when the condition becomes more severe.

Because the lens size is a constant 11.3 mm, a steeper base curve (0.2 mm steeper) as is used to reduce lens movement. However, the biomicroscope is used to observe peripheral clearance and confirm that the peripheral lens area will not adhere to the corneal surface.

The absence of satisfactory peripheral clearance may allow the lens to adhere to the corneal surface. Blinking will induce lacrimal interchange and create various changes in the appearance of the dye patterns in the peripheral areas. However, there may be no visible changes in the apical area for the characteristics of apical clearance.

Silicone elastomer contact lenses seem to settle into their position over time. Consequently, even though the fit may be good, it may be difficult for dye to move behind the lens when it is used to stain the tears. If the patient is instructed to blink hard and to squeeze the lids tightly, the lens fit in the periphery will be loosened so that the dye stained tears can move beneath the lens.

Since silicone elastomer lenses generally sit on the eye in an up-and-out position, dye that appears under the lens edge when the lens is resting on the sclera implies that the lens will not adhere

Figure 8–8. Direct illumination, medium beam, high magnification, showing a mechanically induced corneal abrasion caused by a silicone elastomer contact lens. There is a very narrow band of peripheral clearance, and the lens position is above the geometric center of the cornea. The combination of a poor lens edge finish and lens displacement on blinking has created a mechanical corneal abrasion at the limbus.

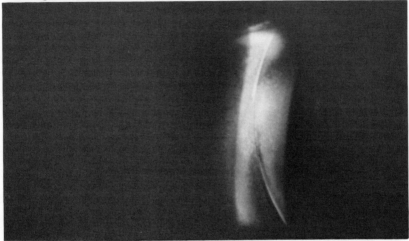

to either the cornea or the scleral surface and that the lens can be removed easily with conventional techniques for either hard or soft contact lenses.

Diffuse illumination, low magnification, is used to observe the apical area. There should be a small amount of apical clearance. Its degree may be reduced on blinking, only to recover after the blink. The action will not create visual distress. This undulating action, described as the *bellows effect,* is believed to be of clinical advantage. On blinking, the upper lid causes a compression of the lens.[3] After blinking, the eye is opened and there is a rapid decompression caused by the high elasticity of the material. The initial volume of tear exchange when the lens is worn is created by motion and bellowing.

The belows effect is progressively reduced as tearing subsides and lens movement decreases. However, a small amount remains, and it assists with the removal of corneal metabolic wastes. Its presence does not preclude wearing comfort.

How to Judge Lens Movement
The practitioner should allow from 10 to 15 minutes for the lens to settle. The fit can be examined sooner if the tearing has obviously subsided.

Lens movement is critical for a successful fit. It should be similar to that of hard corneal lenses, with the lens not moving far from the pupillary area. Blinking should not displace the lens from the cornea, and all movement should be within the corneal area covered by the lens. When the lens extends onto the sclera, lens movement should not disturb the conjunctival or scleral vessels in the area where it rests.

Fluorescein Examination Procedures

There are two categories of dye patterns for silicone elastomer contact lenses: preferred and expected. The preferred dye pattern is an uninterrupted tear-fluorescein film visible behind the lens from edge to edge. The expected, extremely important dye pattern is that of peripheral clearance, having a representative width around the lens circumference. There may be an absence of dye under the peripheral areas where the lens encroaches on the sclera.

1. Use a flatter base curve as a way to increase peripheral clearance. Insufficient clearance will preclude adequate tear interchange beneath the lens. However, the degree of peripheral clearance should not cause the lens edges to lift away from the tears.
2. Use direct illumination, medium beam, low and high magnification, to observe the peripheral fit. Focus the microscope on a peripheral section.
3. When there is an absence of dye under the peripheral curve, instruct the patient to blink very hard once or twice; then observe the fit. Hard blinking will compress the lens and allow more dye to get under it. When the amount of dye under the peripheral curve implies that there is insufficient peripheral clearance, use a new lens with a base curve that is 0.2 mm flatter.

Unlike with a hard corneal lens fit, para-apical corneal bearing is acceptable and indeed is a characteristic of a good fit. Sometimes the practitioner can observe how blinking compresses the lens and moves dye stained tears from under the apical area toward the periphery. This movement confirms that the degree of apical clearance observed will not induce corneal interference. The degree of apical clearance is unacceptable when blinking will not move bubbles away from the apical area toward the periphery. A base curve 0.2 mm flatter should be used to improve the fit.

When there is apical bearing, or a flat fit, there will be an absence of fluorescein in the apical area. There will also be excessive lens movement on blinking, wide peripheral clearance, and possible immobility of the lens on settling. This situation will preclude good lacrimal interchange beneath the lens.

NOTES

1. W. E. Long, "Silicone Rubber Corneal Contact Lenses," in *Symposium on the Flexible Lens: The Future of Flexible Lenses versus Rigid Lenses,* ed. J. L. Bitonte and R. H. Keates (St. Louis: C. V. Mosby, 1972), pp. 73–79.

2. R. H. Hales, "Silicone Lenses," in *Contact Lenses: A Clinical Approach to Fitting,* ed. R. H. Hales (Baltimore: Williams & Wilkins, 1978), pp. 199–204.

3. Ibid.; Long, "Silicone Rubber Corneal Contact Lenses."

Index

Abrasions, corneal, 125–26
  in aphakia, with contact lens
    wear, 39 ff.
  causes of, 182 ff.
  examination for, 69 ff., 200
  with loose lens fit, 217
  phosphatase reaction following,
    185
  recurrent, 183
Adaptation
  abnormal symptoms, 116
  adjustment of corneal metabo-
    lism, 50 ff.
  to all-day wearing, schedule, 176–
    77
  epithelial edema during, 182
  reduction of corneal sensitivity in,
    37
Adler, F. H., 28, 30
Adrian, 39
Aesthesiometer, corneal, 37–38
Allansmith, 143
American Hydron Zero-4 lens, 83,
  84, 87
American Optical Co. Campbell
  biomicroscope, 8, 9, 13
Andrasko, G., 77, 118
Anterior chamber abnormalities,
  seen with conical beam, 2, 65
Aperture fenestrations, 185
Aphakia
  corneal abrasions with contact
    lens wear, 39
  scleral lens fitted for, 54
  surgery, corneal surface pigmen-
    tation from, 169
Apical alignment fitting philosophy,
  214 ff.
Apical bearing
  causing looser lens fit, 218
  fitting philosophy, 214 ff.
  lens, fit too loose centrally, 216

Apical clearance
  fitting philosophy, 214 ff.
  interference with lacrimal inter-
    change, 171–72
  lens producing fit too secure
    centrally, 212 ff.
  minimal, 54
  modification, and lens fit, 196, 215
  reduction of, 167, 198
  restoration of, 198
  in trial lens fit, 82, 202
Aqueous, observation with conical
  beam, 34, 65
Arachnoid corpuscles of corneal
  stroma, 33
Arcuate stains, 124, 127
Arruga, 3
Ashton, N., 29, 41
Astigmatism, corneal, and lens modification, 56
Aubert, 2

Balavoine, C., 34
Basal cells, corneal characteristics
  of, 31, 40
Basal membrane, 32
Base curve
  altered, 200
  in lens design, 83, 162
  modification, 197 ff.
  and lens fit, 202
  relation to peripheral curve, 203
Baud, C. A., 34
Bausch & Lomb
  hydrogel lens, 56, 83–87, 153
  slit lamp, 13
  Thorpe biomicroscope, 9, 13, 160
Bedewing, 32
  conditions indicated by, 176
Bellows effect, 239
Benjamin, B. S., 111
Berens, C., 30

Farinata, corneal, 158
Fatt, I., 29, 79, 117, 120, 121, 122
Feldman, G. L., 99
Flash, electronic, for biomicroscopic
    photography, 16
Fleischer's ring, 70
Fluorescein
    black light examination, 1, 47, 240
    of foreign body lesion, 188
    of too loose fit, 216–17
    of too secure fit, 220
    in examining after lens removal,
        113, 174
    in examining contact lens fit, 5
    in examining for deposits on lens,
        231
    in examining lens/cornea rela-
        tionship, 168
    in localization of corneal insult, 63
    in trial lens fit, 82
    pattern in examination with
        white light, 48
    staining
        in corneal abrasion, 183
        in foreign body lesions, 188
        intracellular, with corneal le-
            sions, 4, 182
        intracellular, in epithelial de-
            nudation, 183
Flynn, W. J., 112
Ford, M. W., 78
Foreign bodies
    causing corneal abrasions, 186
    causing epithelial disturbance,
        175
    on contact lens, 175
    lesions caused by, 188
Francois, J., 27, 30, 31, 32, 33, 34
Freeman, H., 14
Freeman, R. D., 112
Fuch's dystrophy, 2, 158

Glaucoma, 158
Glycogen in corneal epithelium, 31
    with improper contact lens fit, 29
Glycolysis, 28 ff.
Golgi apparatus, 34
Goodlaw, E. I., 73
Grosvenor, T. P., 201
Gullstrand, Allvar, 2, 3, 4, 7, 10
Guttata, corneal, 158

Haag-Streit biomicroscope, 8, 10, 11,
    12, 14, 24, 25, 83
Halo, circumcorneal, 49, 51
Hanna, 40
Hassal-Henle warts, 35
Hathaway, R. A., 97, 102
Henker, 3
Herman, J. P., 114
Hill, R. M., 29, 78, 99, 111, 112
Hirano, J., 29
Holden, B., 35, 132, 134, 138
Holmes, 138
Hruby lens, 2, 7
Hudson-Stahli line, 70
Humphreys, J. A., 134, 138
Hyphaema, 23, 65
Hypopyon, 65
Hypotony, folding of Descemet's
    membrane in, 34
Hypoxia, 122, 128, 141, 214

Illumination
    in biomicroscopic photography, 14
    diffuse
        in examination of anterior cor-
            neal surface, 51
        in examination of lens fit, 53
        in examining bubble formations
            beneath lens, 54
    direct
        classifications, 57–58
        in study of cornea, 56
    in examining for edema, 176
    focal, principle of, 3
    indirect
        in examination of cornea, 69
        in examination of lens charac-
            teristics, 69
    methods in biomicroscopy, 48
    oscillation, technique and uses, 49
    in pre-fitting examination, 155
    proximal, in examination of cor-
        neal and limbal areas, 72
    retro-illumination, 66–70
    sclerotic scatter, 49–51, 166
    slit
        in biomicroscopic photography,
            14, 22
        early development, 1
        specular reflection, 73
    to detect epithelial erosion, 175
    trans-illumination, 66–70